THE EARS NOSE & THROAT

YOUR BODY YOUR HEALTH

THE
EARS
NOSE &
THROAT

Reader's
Digest

The Reader's Digest Association, Inc.

Pleasantville, New York

London Sydney Montreal

The Ears, Nose, and Throat

was created and produced by
Carroll & Brown Limited
20 Lonsdale Road
London NW6 6RD

First English Edition Copyright © 2002

The Reader's Digest Association
LimitedLondon

Copyright © 2003 The Reader's Digest
Association, Inc.

Library of Congress Cataloging-in-Publication Data
Your body your health
   p.cm.
   Includes index.
   Contents: v. 1. The brain and central nervous system.
   ISBN 0-7621-0436-8
   1. Human physiology--Popular works. 2. Human
anatomy--Popular works. 3. Medicine, Popular.
4. Health. I. Reader's Digest Association.

QP38.Y68 2003
613--dc21
                        2002037115
   Contents: v. 5. The Ears, Nose and Throat
   ISBN 0-7621-0469-4

Printed in the United States of America
1 3 5 7 9 6 4 2

IE 004/IC

The information in this book is for
reference only; it is not intended as a
substitute for a doctor's diagnosis and
care. The editors urge anyone with
continuing medical problems or
symptoms to consult a doctor.

American Edition Produced by
NOVA Graphic Services, Inc.
2370 York Road, Suite A9A
Jamison, PA 18929 USA
(215) 542-3900

President
David Davenport

Editorial Director
Robin C Bonner

Composition Manager
Steve Magnin

Associate Project Editor
Linnea Hermanson

Otolaryngology Specialist Consultant
Dr Milan Amin, MD
Drexel University College of Medicine/Hahneman Medical College, Philadelphia

CONTRIBUTORS

Wynnie Chan, BSc, PhD, Public Health Nutritionist

Mr Paul Chatrath, MA (Cantab), MB BS, MRCS, DLO, Specialist Registrar in
Otolaryngology, Royal National Throat, Nose and Ear Hospital, London

Suzy Chiazzari, MIAC, MEDA, MIAHD, MASC, Interior Designer, Stress Consultant and
Colour Therapist

Jayne Comins, MSc, MRCSLT, PG Cert (Voice), Consultant Speech and Language Therapist

Miss Laura Harding, MB BS, FRCS (ORL-HNS), Specialist Registrar in Otolaryngology,
Royal National Throat, Nose and Ear Hospital, London

Dr Lesley Hickin, MB BS, BSc, DRCOG, MRCGP, General Practitioner

Mr Ben Hartley, MB BS, FRCS (ORL-HNS), Consultant Paediatric ENT Surgeon,
Great Ormond Street Hospital for Children, London

Joel Levy, BSc, MA, Medical Writer

Mr S K Lloyd, BSc (Hons), MRCS, Department of Otolaryngology,
Charing Cross Hospital, London

Amanda Sandford, Research Manager, Action on Smoking and Health

Mr David Whinney, FRCS (ORL-HNS), Consultant Ear Nose and Throat Surgeon,
The Royal Cornwall Hospital, Truro

For the Reader's Digest
Editor in Chief Neil E Wertheimer
Art Director Michele Laseau
Senior Designer Judith Carmel
Production Technology Manager Douglas A Croll
Manufacturing Manager John L Cassidy

The Ears, Nose, and Throat

Awareness of health issues and expectations of medicine are greater today than ever before. A long and healthy life has come to be looked on as not so much a matter of luck but as almost a right. However, as our knowledge of health and the causes of disease has grown, it has become increasingly clear that health is something that we can all influence, for better or worse, through choices we make in our lives. *Your Body Your Health* is designed to help you make the right choices to make the most of your health potential. Each volume in the series focuses on a different physiological system of the body, explaining what it does and how it works. There is a wealth of advice and health tips on diet, exercise, and lifestyle factors, as well as the health checks you can expect throughout life. You will find out what can go wrong and what can be done about it, and you will learn from people's real-life experiences of diagnosis and treatment. Finally, there is a detailed A-to-Z index of the major conditions that can affect the system. The series builds into a complete user's manual for the care and maintenance of the entire body.

This volume looks at the interrelated structures and functions of the ears, nose, and throat. Follow a sound from the outside world to the auditory center of your brain and find out why the smell of freshly roasted coffee can evoke memories. Grasp the mechanics of the balance system—and why a rollercoaster ride can leave you literally not knowing which way is up. Find out how to keep your ears, nose, and throat working well and discover how simple self-help measures can help you cope with common infections affecting them. You may be surprised at how easy it is to put your voice under stress and how social habits can adversely affect these delicate organs. Read about what you can do to safeguard ENT (ears, nose, and throat) health against atmospheric threats such as noise and domestic threats such as dust mites. And find out about the ENT specialists, the tests that help them identify problems, and the treatment options available, from drugs to surgery and hearing aids to speech therapy.

Contents

3

What happens when things go wrong

The ENT life story

Your ears, nose, and throat are responsible for much of your communication and interaction with the world around you. The senses of hearing and smell are essential not only to your enjoyment of life and appreciation of the world but also to your very survival. Your throat produces the sounds that enable you to make your thoughts and feelings clear to others.

At first glance, the common link among the ears, nose, and throat is far from obvious, and their primary functions—hearing and balance, smelling, and speaking—may seem widely disparate. But despite the evident differences in their overall structures and functions, these organs and tissues are intimately linked in several ways.

The ears, nose, and throat are anatomically connected by a narrow passage, known as the pharyngotympanic tube. As a result, diseases that affect one will often affect the others, so a single branch of medicine—known as otorhinolaryngology—covers the treatment of all three. They have a developmental connection, because all three derive from similar parts of the fetus, and they share a common degree of sensitivity—the ability to produce or detect incredibly small variations within an extremely wide range of possibilities.

These subtle distinctions are possible because of the delicate and ingenious structures that lie at the heart of each element of the otorhinolaryngeal system.

ENT PRECISION

In the throat, the taut ligaments that make up your vocal cords act like the reed of a musical instrument, giving you the power and precision to produce a range of sounds from a whisper to a song, from a single pure note to the complex articulations that make up language. In the ears, bones and membranes transmit sound waves to pressure-sensitive hairs that translate them into electrical signals with unparalleled sensitivity. Other structures in the ears act like gyroscopes, enabling us to sense gravity and motion and keep our balance. In the nose, millions of receptor cells are alert to odor molecules, producing a device more sensitive than the finest artificial detectors.

THE AQUATIC APE

The complexity and sheer ingenuity of these biological devices is a testament to the power of evolution, although the ancestral roots of some parts of the ears, nose, and throat are surprising. The tiny bones of the middle ears, for instance, evolved from the gill bones of the ancient fish species from which mammals evolved, and according to one controversial theory of human evolution, the specialized human larynx—the lower part of the throat that contains the vocal cords—may have originated as an adaptation to an aquatic lifestyle, rather than in order to facilitate speech.

The "aquatic ape" theory argues that many aspects of human biology indicate that our earliest ancestors (the "missing link" between us and the other types of ape) lived by the sea or large lakes and spent a lot of time immersed in water. According to this theory of evolution, the properties of the human larynx that make speech possible —its length and position in the throat, together with the ability to control breathing voluntarily—first arose in order to help early man take big gulps of air needed for diving. In other words, humans evolved diving apparatuses

A common heritage?

Dolphins and other diving mammals share humans' ability to control breathing voluntarily. Although these animals possess no vocal cords, scientists suggest that certain species of dolphin do produce some sounds in the larynx, although most are made in the nasal sac.

first, and later generations found the adaptations useful to communicate with each other. Evidence from the ear canals of fossil Neanderthal skulls backs up this theory— they sometimes contain bony growths similar to those found in the ears of human divers.

The "aquatic ape" theory is contentious at best. Most evolutionary biologists believe that our ability to articulate words evolved hand in hand with our ability to understand language, one feeding off the other over tens of thousands of years. Child psychologists believe that a similar process is repeated on a much shorter time scale—about four years—every time a child learns to speak.

An especially sensitive nose can distinguish as many as 10,000 separate smells; the average person can detect perhaps half that number.

All in place
The ears, nose, and throat are all visible in the fetus within eight weeks of conception. By five months, these organs are well developed and continue to mature in the womb.

MATURING SENSES

The senses of hearing and smell and the ability to talk all change as you age. Voices deepen, and hearing and smell may become less acute. But if well taken care of, they all make an enormous contribution to your quality of life.

IN THE WOMB

NEWBORN

Musical memory
Recent research suggests that babies are not only able to hear music in the womb but that 12 months later, they show a clear preference for what they heard.

First things first
A baby's throat is designed for simultaneous breathing and breastfeeding, but this means that it lacks the ability to articulate words in the first months of life.

ENT DEVELOPMENT BEFORE BIRTH

Just days after conception, the fertilized human egg has grown into an embryo with a head–tail organization. Within four weeks, six gill-like folds, called "branchial arches," develop at the head end of the embryo. Each arch will become a different set of tissues in the baby—the first two become parts of the ears. Above the arches, at the "top" of the embryo, is a mass of tissue called the fronto-nasal prominence that includes two patches of cells on its surface. These patches will develop into the olfactory lining, where the sense of smell is located. On the outside of the frontonasal prominence is a band of tissue that over the next four weeks curls up and around to form the external nose. By this time, depressions have already formed inside it to produce nostrils.

Meanwhile, below the branchial arches, the beginnings of the digestive system are already present in rudimentary form in the shape of a simple tube. The top of this tube will become the pharynx, and a number of pouches develop from it. The first two pouches link up with the first two branchial arches to give rise to the structures of the ears, including the pharyngotympanic tube, which connects the ears and throat. Meanwhile, a shallow groove in the floor of the primitive pharynx grows into the larynx. Around days 24–26 of development, the nostrils join to the pharynx. By week 8 the fetus has a recognizable face with ears and a nose.

Over the next seven months, these structures develop, fill in, and expand. Some even start functioning. A baby in the womb can hear, for instance, enabling it to recognize

Hearing and listening
Children learn language rapidly, and by the age of five, are using it to hold conversations, ask questions, and listen.

Sound check
As teenagers mature, their voices deepen and becomes more powerful in both boys and girls, with a full range of sounds.

PRESCHOOL

CHILDREN

TEENAGE

Chatter chatter
Toddlers learn words at a phenomenal rate, but their still immature vocal systems mean that their attempts at speaking are not wholly intelligible to others.

Lengthening larynx
At puberty, the larynx becomes longer in boys, resulting in much deeper voices.

its mother's voice at birth. Experts believe that babies may even be able to smell in the uterus, picking up telltale maternal scent molecules in the amniotic fluid, priming them to respond to their mother's odor at birth.

At birth, a newborn baby's vocal apparatus is ready for use, enabling it to scream loudly from its first breath. A newborn, however, lacks the ability to speak, even if it knew how, because its larynx is in the wrong position. For the first six months, the larynx is positioned to allow a baby to breathe at the same time as it breastfeeds.

FROM GURGLES TO RATTLES
In the first six months, babies learn how to integrate the functions of their hearing and speaking apparatuses. At first, they practice making noises—cooing, gurgling, and

laughing for three months, babbling during the following three—while at the same time learning to understand language. By the age of six months babies have a unique ability to distinguish among word sounds they've never heard before, and although they may not speak their first words for another six months, they are already acquiring, with amazing speed, the rules of grammar and syntax that underlie their mother tongue. By the age of three, the average child will be learning 10 new words per day.

During childhood and puberty, the structures of the ears, nose, and throat change and grow. As the skull thickens, the auditory canal connecting the middle ear to the outside world elongates and acquires a slight bend. The eustacian tube doubles in length, making it harder for

Smell the taste
The senses of taste and smell are intrinsically linked, a fact that becomes obvious when we eat: Having a stuffy nose can render food tasteless.

Fragrant flowers
Although the sense of smell becomes less acute in later life, most people retain the ability to discern and enjoy an enormous number of fragrances.

ADULT

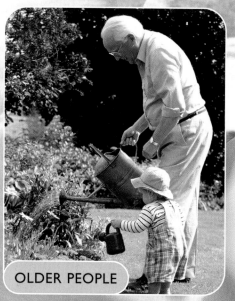

OLDER PEOPLE

bacteria to get from the throat to the ear, so that ear infections become less common. Puberty brings a surge of hormones that affect the vocal cords. The larynx grows and the cords get longer, thicker, and heavier, particularly in males. The average frequency of a child's voice is 265 Hz, for an adult woman it is 225 Hz, and for a man, a low 120 Hz.

While some parts of the ear are growing, however, some are already experiencing the effects of aging. You begin to lose sensory hairs in your inner ear from the moment you are born, causing a very gradual but real decrease in the sensitivity of your hearing. It takes longer for your nose to be affected, but eventually the olfactory sensory cells of the nose begin to thin out, making it harder for older people to detect faint odors and dulling their sense of taste. Even the vocal cords may be affected, stiffening and thinning with extreme old age, so that the voice may become weak. The moment of death itself may be marked by a final spasm of the vocal cords, which produces a "death rattle."

LIFESTYLE AND ENT HEALTH

Day-to-day health issues can also affect the functioning of the vocal cords. A cold can cause swelling and inflammation, leading to hoarseness or even temporary paralysis of the cords. Lifestyle choices such as smoking have a major influence on the incidence and severity of such infections and on the health of other parts of your ears, nose, and throat. Making positive lifestyle choices, including not smoking, avoiding noise and air pollution as much as possible, getting exercise, learning to deal with stress, and adopting a healthy diet, can have profound short- and long-term effects on your otorhinolaryngeal health.

In the long term, a healthy lifestyle can help improve and preserve the sensitivity of your palate and your enjoyment of the subtleties of music and speech, and can be a major contributor to your quality of life. The protective effects of a healthy lifestyle are also important in the short term, because problems affecting your ears, nose, and throat, although not necessarily life-threatening,

The composer Beethoven suffered from the degenerative disease otosclerosis, which today can be treated by surgery or alleviated with a hearing aid.

are among the most irritating and frequently encountered. Ear infections, for instance, are extremely common childhood ailments, which, if poorly managed, can have long-term implications for hearing. Hay fever and other types of allergies are becoming increasingly common, and colds and flu infections are not simply regular nuisances—they pose a real risk to the elderly and vulnerable.

Awareness, a healthy lifestyle, and simple preventative measures can help you to avoid or minimize many ear, nose, and throat problems, and modern medicine has developed a battery of treatments, from the traditional, such as removal of the tonsils, to the advanced, such as cochlear implants ("bionic" inner ear components). Some aspects of ear, nose, and throat medicine have become routine—drug therapies for hay fever, for instance, are now widely available as over-the-counter medicines.

ENT AND THE FUTURE

In the present day, a lot of otorhinolaryngeal medicine focuses on management of problems rather than cures or prevention, but in the future, we may see exciting new avenues of treatment. Short-term prospects include improved cold and flu vaccines, treatments for motion sickness, and radically improved hearing aids.

Further into the future, such technology might be applied to the healthy ear, enhancing normal hearing by selecting what to amplify and what to filter out, helping combat noise pollution. "Smart" hearing aids might even be able to translate normally inaudible sounds or other forms of environmental information into audible sounds. One day you might be able to "hear" your partner's heartbeat or your child's temperature. Similar technology applied in reverse might be used to enhance and alter voices, so that everyone could become an accomplished singer or to modify the sense of smell, so that you could pick up scents that are normally undetectable.

Such bionic senses are a long way off, and many would argue that they are unnecessary for healthy men and women. The human voice is already capable of a fantastic range of expressions, and the amazing structures of your ears and nose have the potential to provide a constantly rich and dazzling sensory feast—as long as you take care of them.

The future of sound
These jagged white waves represent voice patterns produced by a voice-recognition computer. Developments in speech synthesis may help those who have to have their voice boxes removed.

1

How your ears, nose, and throat work

Your amazing ears, nose, and throat

Talking, hearing, smelling, standing upright—these are abilities we usually take for granted. But the structures they depend on are some of the greatest marvels in the human body.

The inner ear *contains the structures needed for hearing and balance. For more information on how they work, see pages 24–25 and pages 26–27.*

The middle ear *contains tiny bones that are so sensitive they can transmit the sound of a pin dropping. Find out how they cope with both loud and soft noises on pages 20–21.*

THE MULTIFUNCTIONAL EARS, NOSE, AND THROAT

Your ears, nose, and throat form an interconnected system of chambers, passages, and extraordinarily complex sensory organs. Among them, these structures perform several major functions—swallowing, the production of sound, balance, hearing, and smell—and a host of minor ones. Smelling, technically known as olfaction, is done by part of the lining of your nasal cavity (the space inside your nose) and your brain. This space opens out into your pharynx and larynx, which together make up your throat, where speech and other sounds are produced. A narrow tube—the eustachian tube—connects the air spaces of your nose and throat to the air spaces of your ear, where the structures of hearing and balance are located. The ear itself has three regions: the outer, middle, and inner ear.

Purposeful pinna
The outer, visible part of your ear is called the pinna. It may not look very useful, but it plays an important role in your hearing; see pages 18–19.

What's in a nose?
The external structure of your nose is made up of skin, bone, and cartilage. Find out how they fit together on pages 28–29.

In the pipeline
The throat is more than a delivery vehicle for food, drink, and air—it also produces sound, enabling you to speak and sing. Turn to pages 34–35 to find out how.

The nose on your face *may be plain to see, but there's a lot that goes on behind it. Find out how the olfactory system works and the roles of the nose, nasal cavities, olfactory lining, and sinuses on pages 30–33.*

The sinuses
Most people's experience of these air-filled cavities is limited to the stuffiness and pain sometimes associated with sinus blockage and fluid during a cold; however, they serve several important functions. See pages 30–31 for more information.

The lining of the nose *is specialized for smelling and also has a defensive role. Find out more on pages 30–33.*

The pharynx and larynx
These two tubes make up the throat. The pharynx runs from the back of the nose to the esophagus. The shorter larynx sits in front and houses the vocal cords. For more information see pages 34–35.

The outer ear

The outer part of the ear performs several important functions without which your hearing would be compromised. It collects sound and directs it to the inner ear, and it helps protect the delicate structures inside the ear from the outside world.

EAR APPARENT

Most of your complex hearing apparatus is hidden away inside your skull, its fragile components shielded by a wall of solid bone. These inner parts are connected to the outside world by a short passage called the auditory or ear canal. The inner end of the canal terminates in a sheet of membrane called the eardrum, and the entrance to the canal is guarded by the visible, outer part of the ear—the pinna.

The sound collector

The pinna, also known as the auricle, is a flap of cartilage and flesh. Apart from providing a physical barrier to foreign objects that might get into the ear, its primary function is to collect sound, in the way that a satellite dish collects television signals, and to direct that sound to the auditory canal.

In men, outer ear tissue continues to grow, so older men have larger pinnae than younger men.

The helix *is the outer curved fleshy ridge of the pinna.*

The concha *is the cavity around which the antihelix curves.*

Auditory canal

The antihelix *is the curved inner ridge of the pinna.*

The mastoid process *is a knob of bone that is the point of attachment for various muscles of the neck.*

Cartilage *runs through the pinna, giving it flexibility and strength.*

The ear lobe *is the fleshy lower part of the pinna.*

Ear exterior
The folds and grooves of the pinna are not there by chance—they modify the transmission of sound waves to the middle and inner ear in a way that helps the brain determine the location of the sound source.

18

Collecting sound
In some ways, the pinna is the reverse of an amphitheater. An amphitheater is designed to amplify sound from the center—the stage —and distribute it so that it can be heard even along the theater's highest rim, whereas the pinna collects sound from the world around it and funnels it toward the middle ear.

The bony parts of the skull
behind the pinna are littered with air spaces.

Eardrum

The auditory canal
The bony parts of the skull behind the pinna are shown in this colored X-ray. The auditory canal that leads to the middle ear is visible at bottom right.

HEARING CANAL

In an adult, the auditory canal is about 1 inch long. The walls of the outer third are made up of flesh and cartilage, whereas the inner two thirds are flesh bound tightly to bone—so tightly that any swelling or inflammation in this zone causes extreme tension and therefore pain. Hairs help prevent large particles from getting into the canal, and glands in the outer part and on the pinna produce wax. There are more than 400 wax glands in each ear. Ear wax traps particles before they can get too far into the canal, helps slow down the growth of bacteria, and protects the canal from becoming waterlogged when water gets into it.

Nerves of the auditory canal

The nerves that supply the auditory canal have the same root as nerves that connect to the airways, stomach, and heart, which is why irritation of the canal, during irrigating or ear cleaning, for instance, can lead to coughing and sneezing and to vomiting in children. The nerves of the auditory canal may be the site of pain from another part of the system, such as a tooth or the tonsils.

The middle ear

The tiny space of the middle ear houses a miniature biological sound system that can outperform any stereo for accuracy of sound reproduction, range of tones, and amplifying power.

DRUM KIT

The middle ear is a space about ⅜ inch wide, ⅜ inch deep, and ⅙ inch high—about the size of a Scrabble tile. Suspended inside this cavity are three bones called the malleus, incus, and stapes, which are collectively known as ossicles (Latin for "little bones"). The role of the ossicles is to transmit sound from the eardrum to the inner ear, where the organs of hearing are located.

FROM AIR TO FLUID

Most of the sound that you hear travels as waves passing through the air. In contrast to the middle ear, the sensory structures of the inner ear sit in fluid. This means that before you can register the sound waves, they have to transfer from air to fluid. Usually, this sort of transfer would result in a loss of energy, making the sound waves much harder to pick up, so the middle ear works to magnify the intensity of sound as it passes from the eardrum, through the ossicles, to the oval window. It does this using a simple trick: The oval window is 22 times smaller than the eardrum, so that the displacement of the eardrum caused by an arriving sound wave is concentrated and thereby magnified 22 times when it is transmitted to the oval window.

BANGING THE DRUM

Your eardrum works like a drum in reverse. With a real drum, a taut sheet of material produces sound waves when struck with a stick. In your eardrum, sound waves from the air strike the taut sheet of membrane, making it vibrate. The vibrations pass to the handle of the malleus, which transmits them to the incus, and then to the stapes. The footplate of the stapes presses down, making the oval window to the inner ear bulge inward.

A NATURAL EQUALIZER

To allow faithful transmission of sound from the eardrum to the oval window, the pressure inside the middle ear must be equal to the pressure in the auditory canal and the rest of the outside world. However, the eardrum makes an airtight seal between the two. To get around this, the middle ear connects to the back of the throat via the 1½ inch long eustachian tube. When you swallow, this tube briefly opens, allowing air to pass in and out of the middle ear and automatically equalizing the pressure on either side of the eardrum.

The ossicles

The three ossicles are individually named in Latin after the tools they resemble: Malleus means hammer, incus is Latin for anvil, and stapes (pictured below) means stirrup. They are the three tiniest bones in the body: The malleus is just ⅓ inch long, and the incus and stapes are of similar size. Our ossicles are descended, via reptilian jaw bones, from the gill bones of primordial fish.

It takes less than one tenth of a second for the muscles attached to the ossicles to tense in reflex to a loud sound.

The malleus *(hammer) bone has a handle, which is attached to the eardrum.*

The incus *(anvil) is attached to the malleus by a freely movable saddle-shaped joint and to the stapes by a ball-and-socket joint.*

Overload protection system
The ossicles have to be extremely sensitive to pick up very faint sounds, but this makes them vulnerable to damage from loud noises. The tensor tympani and stapedius muscles that attach to the ossicles help prevent this damage by tensing when a loud noise occurs. The muscles' tensing limits the movement of the ossicles, damping down strong vibrations to safe levels.

The oval window *is sealed by a flexible membrane around the stapes that forms a barrier between the middle ear and the beginning of the cochlea within the inner ear.*

The stapes *(stirrup) has a bony footplate that sits on the oval window.*

The round window *is sealed by a flexible membrane. It divides the middle ear and the other end of the cochlea.*

The eardrum *is oval and about ⅓ inch high, and it bulges slightly into the tympanic cavity. It is also called the tympanic membrane.*

The eustachian tube *leads from the middle ear to the throat.*

Examining the eardrum
A colored scanning electron micrograph (SEM) shows the eardrum and two of the three ossicles: the malleus and the incus.

The inner ear

On either side of your skull—about 1⅗ inches from the outside—are the bony labyrinths, where the energy of sound waves, gravity, or head movements is translated into nervous impulses for your brain to interpret.

ENTER THE LABYRINTH

The inner ear's bony labyrinth is a series of tubes that coil and interconnect. Inside this hard shell, following its twists and turns, is a set of fluid-filled, tube-shaped, membranous sacs called the membranous labyrinth. Inside the membranous labyrinth are the structures that translate input such as the direction of gravity or the frequency of a sound wave into nerve impulses. The bony labyrinth has three main components: the vestibule, the semicircular canals, and the cochlea.

HAIRS OF HEARING

The three parts of the inner ear use different structures to perform their varied sensory tasks, but all rely on the same underlying mechanism—the translation of physical movement into a nerve impulse. This is performed by hair cells, which are found in all three parts of the inner ear. A hair cell is a specialized sensory cell. At the top of the hair cell, tiny hairs called stereocilia and kinocilia stick out. At its base, the hair cell connects to the nervous system. Movement of the hairs, such as that caused by a passing sound wave, causes chemical changes in the cell membrane surrounding the hair. These changes in turn cause the hair cell to fire off a nerve impulse from its base.

The bony labyrinths
The location of the bony labyrinths within a human skull are shown above. The outline of the outer ears can be seen on either side, with the nose at the top.

Inside the cochlea
A computed tomography (CT) scan reveals an interior cross section through one turn of the cochlea.

Liquid center

The membranous labyrinth is filled with a type of fluid called endolymph and surrounded by a different fluid called perilymph. Endolymph has special properties that enhance the sensitivity of the hair cells. It contains high levels of electrolytes, which cause the hair cells to be more easily triggered by tiny movements.

The bony labyrinth *surrounds the membranous labyrinth and the structures that lie within: the vestibule, the semicircular canals, and the cochlea.*

Anterior semicircular canal

Lateral semicircular canal

Perilymph *surrounds the membranous labyrinth.*

The membranous labyrinth *of the vestibule and semicircular canals is more or less continuous, so they are sometimes collectively referred to as the vestibular complex.*

Posterior semicircular canal

Ampullae—*swellings in the semicircular canals filled with endolymph—are the location of the sensory cells that detect head movement.*

The three semicircular canals *sense the force and direction of head movements, thus helping you balance.*

Oval window

Stapes

The vestibule *senses gravity, telling you which way is up.*

The vestibular nerve *leads to the vestibulocochlear nerve, which travels to the brain.*

Round window

The cochlear nerve *is also a branch of the vestibulocochlear nerve.*

Cochlea

Eustachian tube

The cochlea *detects the tone and loudness of incoming sound waves, providing your sense of hearing. By comparing the timing and strength of signals from the cochleas on either side of your head, your brain can determine the location of a sound source.*

Hearing

The cochlea, within the inner ear, contains the hearing apparatus that is able to sense the two defining aspects of sound—frequency, also known as pitch, and loudness, also known as amplitude.

SURROUND SOUND

The cochlea is a bony coil with two-and-a-half turns. It begins at the oval window and ends at the round window; the end of the coil farthest away from these windows is called the apex. The cross section shows that the cochlea is made up of three ducts. The top and bottom (vestibular and tympanic) ducts are filled with perilymph; they join up at the cochlea's apex, so that they actually comprise a single continuous duct that starts at the oval window and finishes at the round window. The middle duct is called the cochlear duct; this is filled with endolymph and contains the Organ of Corti, where sound sensing takes place.

SOUND DETECTION

Loudness is determined by the amount of bending and flexing that sensory stereocilia undergo. The frequency (pitch) that you hear is determined by which part of the cochlea vibrates (or resonates) most in response to an incoming sound. Lower frequency sounds resonate most at the apex of the cochlea; higher frequencies resonate at the cochlea's base, near the cochlear nerve. The different regions of the cochlea map directly onto the part of the brain that interprets sound, so that a signal from the apex of the cochlea is translated into the sensation of hearing a low-frequency sound.

There are more than a million sensory hairs (stereocilia) in the cochlea.

From middle ear to inner ear
Sound waves trigger the vibration of the footplate of the stapes bone against the flexible membrane covering the oval window.

Oval window

Stapes

1 *Sound waves are funneled by the outer ear into the auditory canal and toward the eardrum. The sound waves make the eardrum vibrate, which in turn causes all three ossicles to vibrate.*

2 *When the footplate of the vibrating stapes presses down against the oval window, the oval window bulges inward, and sound waves are transmitted through the oval window to the perilymph-filled ducts in the cochlea.*

Bony cochlear wall

Vestibular duct

Reissner's membrane *separates the vestibular duct from the cochlear duct.*

The Organ of Corti
This essentially consists of rows of sound-sensing hair cells attached to a basilar membrane. The stereocilia projecting from the top of the hair cells are attached to a tectorial membrane that forms a rooflike structure above them.

Tectorial membrane

Hair cell topped by stereocilia

Organ of Corti within the cochlear duct

Tympanic duct

Cochlear nerve

Basilar membrane

Nerve fiber leading to the cochlear nerve

Auditory cortex within the temporal lobe

Brain

Cochlear apex

Round window

Vestibulocochlear nerve

Location of the cochlear nucleus of the medulla

Cochlear base

3 *As waves pass along the cochlea, they set the Organ of Corti's basilar membrane vibrating, while the Organ of Corti's tectorial membrane stays put. This causes the stereocilia at the top of the hair cells between the two membranes to bend and flex.*

4 *Displacement of the cilia triggers each hair cell to fire off a nerve signal down the cochlear nerve. The cochlear nerve joins the vestibular nerve to form a bundle of fibers making up the vestibulocochlear nerve, which leads to the brain.*

5 *Nerve impulses carried along the vestibulo-cochlear nerve enter the brain at the cochlear nucleus of the medulla and are sent to the auditory cortex of the temporal lobe, where they are interpreted.*

25

Balance

Normally, you only notice your sense of equilibrium when it's not right. But underlying this sense is a remarkable marriage of basic mechanical principles and complex, high-precision, biological engineering.

MAKING SENSE OF MOTION

In order to be able to stand up, sit down, and walk around, never mind more complex maneuvers such as handstands, your body needs to be able to sense a number of different things: the direction of gravity, your orientation with respect to gravity, and the speed and angle of movement of your head (which controls the rest of the body). All these components contribute to your overall sense of balance.

It is the semicircular canals (in the inner ear's bony labyrinth) that allow you to sense the motion of your head. Each ear has three canals, at right angles to each other, so you can sense movement in any plane.

DETECTING HEAD MOVEMENT

Inside the ampulla of each of your inner ear's semicircular canals is a structure called the crista. The crista is made up of hair cells on the wall of the ampulla. Tiny cilia (kinocilia and stereocilia) at the top of these hairs are embedded in a gelatinous mass called the cupula, which floats in the endolymph. When your head moves, the inertia of the cupula makes it lag slightly behind, so that it tugs on the cilia and activates the hair cells. When your head stops, the cupula overshoots slightly, tugging on the cilia in the other direction. The movement of the cilia in any direction triggers nerve impulses, which are then interpreted by the brain.

A cross section of a crista *and cupula in the inner ear. The crista is the sensory structure that detects head movement.*

Endolymph

The cupula *is a gelatinous mass.*

Cilia *protrude from the crista into the cupula.*

Hair cell

Supporting cell
Sensory nerve

Cilia are upright when the head is still.

The cupula tugs the cilia sideways as the head stops turning.

Turning sideways
When the head moves from side to side—as here— or backward or forward, so do hair cells in the inner ear's semicircular canals. Shifting hair cells trigger nerve impulses that keep the brain informed of the head's exact position.

Limestone in your ears
A scanning electron microscope reveals the structure of a single otolith. Otoliths are made out of calcium carbonate, which is also found in limestone, chalk, and marble.

Taking a bow
As the head bends forward—as here— backward, or sideways, sensory hair cells of the inner ear's vestibule follow suit. This allows your brain to detect the pull of gravity when you move your head.

SENSING THE PULL OF GRAVITY

Hair cells in the vestibule component of the inner ear provide your sense of gravity. They are found in clusters called maculae within the saccule and the utricle—both parts of the membranous labyrinth inside the vestibule. As with hair cells of the semicircular canals, the cilia are embedded in a gelatinous mass, but in this case there is an added ingredient—millions of tiny mineral crystals called otoliths. Their weight provides a mass for gravity to work on. When you are standing upright, gravity presses them down, slightly squashing the cilia on the hair cells, which triggers the production of nerve impulses. If you tilt your head, the mass of otoliths slides to one side, pulling the cilia with them and sending matching nerve impulses to the brain.

Endolymph

Cilia (stereocilia and kinocilia) *are embedded in the gelatinous mass.*

A layer of otoliths *sits on top of a gelatinous mass.*

Hair cell

Supporting cell

Sensory nerve

Cilia are upright when the head is upright.

Cilia bend downward as the head drops forward.

A cross section of a macula *within the vestibule. The macula is the sensory structure that detects the pull of gravity.*

The nose

The visible part of your respiratory and olfactory systems is your nose. Big or small, it protects the entrance to your airways and helps you gather samples of air to smell.

FLESH AND BONES

The external nose is a covering of skin and flesh over a supporting framework of bone and cartilage. Pieces of cartilage provide the stiff framework that prevents the nostrils from collapsing. The inside of the nose is divided in two by the nasal septum.

NO NOSE IS BAD NOSE

The external nose serves a number of important functions.

- The cartilage and bone keep the nostrils open for easy passage of air, and nostril hairs and the ability to narrow the nostrils in response to an offensive odor (that is, wrinkle your nose) help prevent noxious gases or foreign objects from getting into the respiratory system.
- By effectively extending the respiratory and olfactory tract beyond the face, the nose allows you to sample smells from inside objects or through narrow openings—in other words, you can poke your nose into places the face cannot fit.
- Lastly, and perhaps most obviously, your nose prevents water from running into your breathing passages by shielding them from the rain, like an umbrella, or by trapping air (and thereby keeping out the water) if you need to submerge your head.

CARTILAGE AND BONE

The nasal bones *project slightly from the front of the skull. They are fused to the maxilla (the facial bone).*

Lateral cartilage *extends from the nasal bones to form the more flexible part of your nose.*

The alar cartilages *form wings of cartilage that flank the outer edges of the nostrils.*

The accessory cartilages *lie between the lateral part of the alar cartilage and the bony nasal opening.*

Crucial underpinning
Bone and cartilage work together to provide the framework that enables the nose to perform its main function of allowing air to enter through the nostrils.

Made for smelling
Because the nose projects from the face, it can catch subtle scents that might otherwise be missed.

INSIDE THE NOSE

LOOKING UP THE NOSTRILS

Nasal hairs *help keep out unwanted visitors, including insects, pollen, dirt, and other material.*

Alar cartilage

Septal cartilage

The frontal process *(meaning prominence) of the maxilla.*

Lateral cartilage

Nostril

The septal cartilage *forms the barrier between the two nostrils.*

The alveolar process *(prominence) of the maxilla.*

The maxilla— *the main facial bone—surrounds the nose on both sides and below.*

The lining of the two nostrils
The nostrils' lining is covered with a very delicate membrane, rich in blood vessels and nerve endings. This can be painful if it is damaged and tends to bleed easily.

The nares— *the openings to the nostrils—are surrounded by fibrofatty tissue, which overlays the greater alar cartilages.*

Vertical cross section of the nose
The projecting parts of the nose have been cut away to reveal the nostrils and septal cartilage.

Skin protection
The vulnerable, exposed outer skin of the nose is well supplied with tiny sebaceous glands. These secrete oil to provide a protective oily coating for the skin that keeps the skin supple and forms a barrier between the skin and the air outside.

Research has found that the nose may swell slightly and lengthen as a result of the stress induced by telling a lie.

The nasal cavity

Between the roof of your mouth and the bottom of your brain is an irregularly shaped space known as the nasal cavity, which has important roles in respiration, smell, and defending the body from illness.

THE NASAL CAVITY

The front of the nasal cavity is connected to the outside world by the nostrils, and at the back it opens onto the top of the throat. Several smaller chambers, called sinuses, lead off from the sides. The nasal cavity's functions include olfaction (sense of smell); filtering, heating and humidifying incoming air to prevent damage to the lungs; and defense against invading micro-organisms. The cavity is mostly lined with a moist mucous membrane that produces mucus and is equipped with cilia to help carry "dirty" mucus to the throat, where it is swallowed. In addition, the olfactory lining on the roof of the nasal cavity includes sensory receptors that respond to odor molecules, providing your sense of smell.

THE PARANASAL SINUSES

Because the various sinuses adjacent to the nasal cavity are usually filled with air, they provide resonant spaces that are important in the production of sound. Their extensive inner surfaces are lined with a mucus-producing membrane, so they can generate large amounts of mucus for flushing out the nasal cavity.

The great divide
In mammals, the nasal cavity and the mouth are divided by the palate, separating the digestive and olfactory systems. This allows mammals to use their sense of smell even while their mouths are full—a vital skill for prey animals such as antelope, which need to be on guard at all times.

Side view of the nasal cavity
The air-filled nasal cavity is divided vertically down the middle by the bone and cartilage septum.

Frontal sinus

Ethmoidal sinus

The sphenoidal sinus *is an air-filled cavity, as are all the paranasal sinuses.*

Concha

Septum

The nasopharynx *is the upper part of the pharynx, above the level of the soft palate. It is connected to the nasal cavity.*

Bony part of the palate

Soft part of the palate
This is the part of the palate that is pushed up when you swallow, closing the nasal cavity off from the mouth and preventing food from going up the back of the nose.

When you breathe
The soft palate is relaxed, allowing air inhaled via the mouth to move freely into the nasopharynx and the nasal cavity.

When you swallow
The soft palate moves up to form a barrier between the pharynx and the nasal cavity so that food cannot get into the nasal cavity.

The conchae

Also known as the turbinate bones, the conchae are bony protrusions into the nasal cavity designed to interrupt the flow of incoming air and cause turbulence. Incoming air bounces around in the nasal cavity, picking up heat and moisture and depositing dust and germs in the mucus that lines the cavity.

The paranasal sinuses

The paranasal sinuses include two frontal cavities, two maxillary cavities, and two anterior ethmoidal sinuses (which consist of many spaces within the ethmoid bone). There are also two sphenoidal sinuses and the two posterior ethmoidal sinuses, which are positioned too far back in the head to be shown here.

Left and right frontal sinuses

Superior meatus
The meatuses are the channels between the conchae.

Superior concha

Anterior ethmoidal sinus

Middle meatus

Middle concha

Inferior meatus

Maxillary sinus

Maxilla

Inferior concha

The septum *is bony at the back of the nose and composed of cartilage at the front.*

The nasal cavity includes between 10 and 20 million smell receptors, all found within the olfactory region that forms part of the lining of the cavity roof.

Cross section of the nasal cavity

The nasal cavity and paranasal sinuses are connected by narrow passages, so that air can enter the sinuses from the nasal cavity and mucus manufactured in the sinuses is transported the other way into the nasal cavity and then swallowed.

Smell

Smell is one of the most sensitive and powerful of the primary senses, producing emotional reactions and associations thanks to its unique connections with the brain. It is often underrated and underused by humans.

THE OLFACTORY REGION

Every time you breathe in, air flows around your nasal cavity between the ridges and bumps of the nasal conchas. About 2 percent of this inhaled air passes over the olfactory region at the top of the nasal cavity that provides your sense of smell (olfactory sense). This olfactory region is rich in sensory receptor cells that sample odor molecules carried on the air; if triggered, they fire off nerve signals to the brain. The olfactory region is unusual in that it connects directly to the brain; this may account for the emotions, memories and associations that a smell can trigger.

Olfactory receptor cells *are modified nerve cells. A long axon carries nerve signals from the base of each receptor cell into the olfactory bulb and toward the brain.*

Supporting cells *are believed to help clear away unwanted odor molecules that might confuse or swamp the receptor cells. They are covered in tiny hairs called microvilli, which increase their surface area and so makes them more effective.*

The olfactory bulb *is an outgrowth of the brain itself. There are two bulbs— one on each side of the septum, which divides the nasal cavity in two.*

Axon

Olfactory bulb

Bone

Mucus glands

Apical knob

Cilia within mucus

The olfactory region within the nasal cavity *is an area of yellowish membrane about the size of a postage stamp.*

The olfactory tract *connects the brain to the olfactory bulb.*

Bone

Superior nasal concha

Olfactory region of the nasal cavity

Nasal cavity

Soft palate

Hard palate

Smelling step by step

Olfaction is carried out by specialized receptor cells. These are essentially nerve cells with long hairs called cilia projecting from one end.

1. Odor molecules carried in the air pass over the olfactory region within the nasal cavity.
2. The odor molecules dissolve in the mucus that lines the nasal cavity.
3. The molecules reach receptor cells specialized to respond to their particular odor and bind to receptor molecules on the surface of the receptor cell, triggering a response.
4. The receptor cell sends a nerve signal to the brain.

Apical knob: *Each receptor cell is capped with a raised apical knob that projects very slightly through the surface of the olfactory region.*

Cilia: *Sprouting out of each apical knob are around 10 to 20 whiplike filaments called cilia, each 0.0001 mm wide. Cilia increase the surface area to which odor molecules can bind.*

Odor molecule *dissolved in the mucus that lines the nasal cavity.*

Odor molecule *carried along within inhaled air.*

Close-up of a single apical knob
This scanning electron micrograph shows an apical knob—the yellow patch at bottom right—with cilia radiating from its surface.

THE JOURNEY FROM THE NOSE TO THE BRAIN

Axons projecting from the base of each receptor cell join into nerve bundles. These travel through the bone that separates the nasal cavity from the brain and connect to the olfactory bulb—an outgrowth of the brain itself. From here, nerves connect directly to the brain's cortex, where olfactory information is processed. This means that smells are the only sensations to reach the cortex without having to go through the thalamus, a lower brain structure that normally filters and processes incoming information. In addition, the olfactory bulb has direct connections to the brain's limbic system and hippocampus, parts of the brain that are involved in memory and emotion.

Limbic system

Thalamus

Cerebral cortex

Nerve pathway

Frontal lobe

Olfactory bulb

Air and odor molecules being inhaled

Larynx

The throat and sound production

Leading from the back of the nasal cavity to the top of the trachea and the entrance to the esophagus, your throat is involved in the key processes of digestion, respiration, and speech, or phonation.

The vocal cords are so elastic, they can be stretched by as much as half their length again.

TOUR OF THE THROAT

The throat is made up of the pharynx and the larynx. The pharynx is a 4½–5½ inch long muscular tube that leads from the nose and mouth to the top of the esophagus—the pipe that carries food to the stomach. An opening called the glottis leads into the larynx, a cartilaginous tube that contains the vocal cords and protects the entrance to the trachea, down which air travels to the lungs. The average laryngeal length is 1⅘ inches in men but only 1⅗ inches in women.

TONSILS AND ADENOIDS

Both tonsils and adenoids are made up of collections of immune cells called lymphocytes that form centers of defense against invading microorganisms. You'll find the tonsils at the far back and sides of your mouth, within the oropharynx. The adenoids are situated high in the back of the throat behind the nose and the roof of the mouth, in the nasopharynx.

The pharynx *extends in its entirety from the back of the nose to the top of the esophagus. It has three parts: the nasopharynx, the oropharynx, and the laryngopharynx.*

The nasopharynx *runs from the nasal cavity to the soft palate.*

Soft palate

Body of the tongue

The oropharynx *lies between the soft palate and the glottis.*

The glottis *is the opening of the larynx, which contains the vocal cords.*

The epiglottis *is a hinged piece of cartilage that protects the glottis. When you swallow, it swings down to cover the glottis, preventing food or liquid from entering the trachea and lungs.*

Vocal cords

The thyroid cartilage *is the largest piece of cartilage in the larynx. It is also called the Adam's apple.*

The larynx—*commonly known as the voice box—is made up of several pieces of cartilage held together with ligaments. It runs from just below the epiglottis to the beginning of the trachea.*

The laryngopharynx *runs from the glottis to the esophagus.*

The esophagus *begins at the base of the neck, just below a ring of cartilage called the cricoid.*

The trachea *starts just below the crichid cartilage.*

MAKING SOUND

Like any sound production system, the voice box needs three basic components.

An energy source Your breath provides the energy for sound production.

An oscillator Your vocal cords and the space between them act as an oscillator. By vibrating very quickly—up to 250 times per second—the cords set up a series of oscillations in the air stream (in the same fashion as a siren). These determine the basic pitch of the sound.

A resonator Resonation of the vocal cords adds harmonics, without which speech is unintelligible. Your larynx, pharynx, and oral and nasal cavities make up your vocal tract, which holds a column of air that acts as a flexible resonator. You can adjust the length, volume, shape, and tension of the tract to filter out some of the pitches and harmonics produced by the vocal cords, and amplify and add to others.

Sound bites

The pitch and harmonics produced by your voice box provide the basic vowel sounds of speech, but the addition of consonants and the way that both vowels and consonants are "articulated" (shaped and combined) depend on the action of your tongue, palate, lips, cheeks, and teeth.

THE VOCAL CORDS

The vocal cords are highly elastic ligaments strung across the larynx with folds or flaps of tissue attached. At the back of the larynx, they attach to fingers of mobile cartilage. When you speak, the muscles of your larynx twist and move these fingers, stretching and flexing the vocal cords in turn. The longer the vocal cords are, the lower their resonant frequency and the deeper the voice produced. It is because the male vocal cords lengthen at puberty that boys' voices change and become deeper.

Open and relaxed

Closed and taut

Cartilage Glottis Epiglottis Ventricular fold Vocal cord, *also known as a vocal fold.*

During normal breathing *the vocal cords are relaxed and open. When you speak or sing, they become more or less taut.*

The ventricular folds *are flaps of tissue that close off the glottis when you swallow and protect the vocal cords. They are also called the false vocal cords.*

A day in the life of your ears, nose, and throat

Your ears, nose, and throat are highly responsive to changes in both the external and internal environment. Conscious control, involuntary reflexes, and chemical messengers combine to fine tune their day-to-day functioning.

Taking time out
Playing with your sense of balance on the rides at a fair or theme park can be fun. A rollercoaster ride sends the otoliths within the vestibule of your inner ear into free fall, because your head is pulled back and forth by the fierce tug of gravity.

HOME AND AWAY

Your ears, nose, and throat are controlled by a combination of nerve signals from the brain and local control mechanisms. The ear, for example, can protect itself against damage from loud noises with the help of feedback from the brain, and the mucous lining of the sinuses responds to signals from local immune tissues. Your ears, nose, and throat also help control other systems of your body, such as head orientation and facial muscle action.

8:00 A.M. Nasal intelligence

As you head for the kitchen for breakfast you realize that your partner has the coffee on already—your nostrils flare to capture more of the rich aroma and suddenly you remember the Parisian café where you ate breakfast as a student. Your reverie is interrupted by a less pleasant smell: As you become aware that the toast is burning, signals are sent to the facial muscles around your nose, stimulating them to contract and producing a wrinkling of the nose. This narrows the nostrils and prevents more odor molecules from getting in.

8:45 A.M. Under pressure

On your journey to work, the train enters a tunnel. This causes the air pressure around you to increase, but the air in your middle ear is still at the same pressure as before. This produces a feeling of discomfort and prevents the accurate transmission of sound waves through the ossicles, so that everything sounds dulled. You swallow, causing your larynx to rise and your pharynx to contract. This opens the end of the eustachian tube, letting air into your middle ear, equalizing the pressure and enabling you to hear normally again.

10:00 P.M. Time to relax—and rest

The day is drawing to a close and all you want to do is unwind before going to bed. You draw a deep bath, into which you pour some bubblebath and a few drops of your favorite aromatherapy oil. As you lie back and take the first of a series of slow, relaxing breaths, the bath oil begins to work its magic. Soothing vapors are gently sucked into your nasal cavity, where the aroma is picked up by sensory receptor cells in the olfactory region on the roof of the nasal cavity. From here, nerve signals to the olfactory bulb in the brain trigger feelings of peace, pleasure, and letting go—a fitting end to the day.

5:00 P.M. Keeping your balance

You head for the gym after work, and as you lunge up, down, forward and sideways, it is your sense of balance that saves you from falling flat on your face. Tiny cilia attached to hair cells within the semicircular canals and vestibule of your inner ear move in the same direction as your head. The resulting nerve signals allow you to maintain a precise awareness of the speed and angle of your head—key knowledge when it comes to controlling the movement of your body.

1:00 P.M. Volume control

There's a lot of drilling at a building site next to the office, which sends blasts of very loud sound waves into your ear, causing large movements of the hairs in your ear's cochlea. A nerve signal races toward your brain stem (where the brain meets the spinal cord) and triggers a reflex feedback signal to the muscles attached to your ossicles within the middle ear. The muscles contract, dampening the excessive and potentially damaging vibrations of the ossicles and thereby also protecting your cochlear receptor hairs. At the same time, another reflex nerve signal from the brain stem activates your neck muscles, turning your head so you face the source of the sound.

2

Keeping your ears, nose, and throat healthy

CARING FOR THE EARS, NOSE, AND THROAT

The ears, nose, and throat are in constant contact with outside stimuli, and much of the time they function without us being aware of them, but problems in one area may affect the others.

 41 *Understanding how your ears, nose, and throat work, and the relationship among them, is the first step to good health.*

 44 *Simple good habits in your daily life can help to achieve a lifetime of good health for your ears, nose, and throat.*

 46 *The senses of hearing, smell, and taste change as we age. Knowing the changes to expect enables you to seek help for problems early on.*

 51 *Common symptoms affect the ears, nose, and throat often, so it is important to know when to ignore and when to treat them.*

 54 *Understanding how infections of the ears, nose, and throat are spread will enable you to treat them swiftly and effectively.*

 55 *Both pharmacists and complementary therapists have a wealth of remedies to treat common ENT ailments.*

 59 *Being a wise traveler can help you to avoid motion sickness and other potential problems of the ears, nose, and throat.*

Understanding your ENT

Learning how your ears, nose, and throat function independently from one another and how they are related gives you the information you need to sense when your ENT health might be changing for the worse.

YOUR EARS AND HEARING

Of the five senses, hearing probably does the most in helping you communicate with the world around you. Your ears are simply amazing, allowing you to enjoy a Beethoven recital, join in a conversation, or hear a police siren. If your ears are functioning correctly, this usually happens unconsciously.

It is only when you concentrate on a specific sound that you become aware of using your sense of hearing. Your ears not only perceive sounds of very low and very high pitches but are also able to detect varying intensities of sound. The sounds that you hear are a result of many single frequencies being integrated into a tone by your brain.

We all take our hearing for granted, and, quite often, hearing loss can go undetected for some time, particularly if it is gradual or in only one ear. If you are concerned about the quality of your hearing, there are several questions you can ask yourself to ascertain whether you have a problem (see page 52).

Dual signals

Most sounds can be distinguished perfectly well with one ear alone. The task of pinpointing where a sound comes from, however, is dependent on both ears. The brain interprets the subtle differences in data from each ear and combines them. Pattern recognition can tell us whose voice we are hearing or what car is arriving. The human ear is so specialized that not only can we recognize the similarities among sounds so that words are heard, but we can also detect enough to know exactly who is speaking.

Sound overload
Your ears have to detect thousands of different sounds every day and then pass on this information to your brain, which interprets what those sounds are and prepares your body for a response.

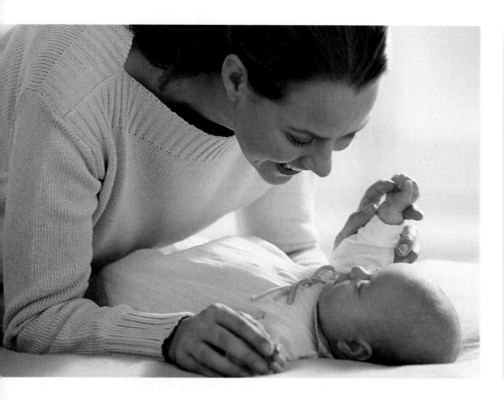

Unique scent

In one study, babies as young as six weeks old correctly identified their own mother's T-shirt by scent.

KEEPING YOUR BALANCE

Staying upright is governed by your inner ear. It responds to your head's movement and position relative to gravity and triggers a response in the brain to restore the equilibrium. The inner ear needs help, however, and balance relies to a considerable extent on the eyes as well. They send similar messages to the brain based on movement. Your sense of balance is challenged when the messages from the inner ear and the eyes differ —often during times of high speed and motion, such as on a rollercoaster.

A NORMAL NOSE

You rely on your sense of smell for more information about your surroundings than you probably realize. It is important in all animal behavior, for identification of food, mates, and predators. For humans, it also provides sensual pleasure, as well as warning of dangers such as spoiled food and escaping gas.

Are you led by your nose?

Perfume companies try to tell us that wearing their products will instantly make us more sexually attractive. However, studies have indicated that we have our own smell-signaling system. Chemicals called pheromones may partly govern our sexual identification and behavior.

In humans, the most important odor-producing organ is the skin. The skin's apocrine glands produce substances detectable only by the human nose. However, there is another scent detection system, located on the nasal septum, that may also detect these chemicals.

Scientists have demonstrated that by six weeks of age a baby can differentiate its own mother's smell.

In addition, it has been observed since the 1960s that, under the influence of pheromones, women living in the same house tend to have their period at around the same time of month. Young adults can distinguish their own scent from others and can also differentiate male from female body odor on clothing.

Sweet smelling

From as far back as Roman days, people have worn scent to make themselves more sexually attractive.

THE THROAT

Your throat contains two important areas of immune cells called the tonsils and adenoids. In children, these are important at fighting off respiratory tract and lung infections, but they can become so enlarged that they interfere with the functioning of the ears, nose, and throat. Following adolescence, they become unnecessary and shrink and few adults are aware of their presence.

At the base of your throat lies the larynx—yet another part of your ears, nose, and throat involved in communication. When functioning poorly, the larynx displays signs of hoarseness or loss of voice, which you will experience as a "sore" throat.

INTERRELATED SYSTEMS

Your ears, nose, and throat are closely related both in terms of structure and function. A problem in any one of these organs can spread to or produce symptoms in another. Not only are the three connected, they all produce warm fluid—a perfect medium for bacteria and viruses to multiply.

An infection in the nose or throat can easily spread to the ears or to the paranasal sinuses, which become blocked by fluid. An ear infection may cause balance problems, and enlarged adenoids can block the eustachian tube, causing pain in the ear and the nose, making breathing difficult. Conversely, an obstruction in the nasal space can block ears.

A blocked eustachian tube can also occur during a bad cold or hay fever and produce pain when swallowing and fluid in the middle ear.

Colds and hay fever can produce symptoms in all these organs, either all at once or one after another.

WELL CONNECTED

The interrelationship of your ears, nose, and throat explains why discomfort or infection in one part of the system may easily spread to another. All are connected in more ways than one, with some perhaps surprising parts of the ENT system directly joined. The labels below identify the most important connections.

NOSE—SINUSES
The nose is connected to the paranasal sinuses, which drain fluid into the nose.

NASAL CAVITY—PHARYNX
The nasal cavity is connected to the nasopharynx.

EARS—THROAT
The ears are connected directly to the throat by the eustachian tube, which opens and closes to allow air to enter the middle ear, keeping it at atmospheric pressure.

EARS—THROAT
The eustachian tube also carries mucus produced in the middle ear to the throat, where it can be swallowed.

THROAT—ESOPHAGUS
The throat connects the mouth and esophagus. During swallowing, food is directed down the esophagus.

THROAT—TRACHEA
The throat is connected to the trachea, where air passes on its way to and from the lungs.

The ears, nose, and throat in daily life

Your ears, nose, and throat are constantly bombarded by pollutants, viruses, bacteria, pollen, alcohol, noise, air pressure ...the list is endless. How your body reacts to irritants can have an effect on your day-to-day activities and well-being.

When they are working well, you are likely to be almost unaware of your ears, nose, and throat. Several everyday situations have an impact on them, however. Knowing when they might be compromised enables you to take sensible precautions to preserve your health.

PREVENT EAR INFECTIONS

Acute earaches are usually the result of an infection in the inner ear, most often caused by the bacteria or viruses from a cold or the flu traveling along the eustachian tube and settling there. The infection stimulates an increase in secretion from the mucous membranes but often, the eustachian tube is so inflamed by the infection that the fluids are unable to drain. The structure of the eustachian tube in children allows viruses and bacteria to reach the middle ear much more frequently, with a greater risk of infection. The adenoids are relatively larger in children than in adults and can press on the opening to the eustachian tube, which can prevent mucus or fluid from draining out of the middle ear and increase the risk of an ear infection.

Poorly functioning eustachian tubes can cause the sensation of muffled hearing and pain. In severe cases, the eardrum may perforate.

HOW TO BLOW YOUR NOSE

Believe it or not, there is a right way and a wrong way to blow your nose. If you apply too much pressure, you risk forcing harmful bacteria into your sinus cavities or ears or even

Depressurize
The rapid drop in pressure during a sky dive presents serious risk to the ears—during a jump it is vital to equalize the pressure in your ears to prevent damage.

rupturing an eardrum. The best advice is to blow one nostril at a time while pressing gently on the other one. Blow frequently to prevent mucus buildup and use a tissue. A dab of petroleum jelly around the nostrils may help to prevent soreness.

CHANGING PRESSURE

Air is usually able to pass freely into the middle ear to maintain atmospheric pressure. Under certain circumstances, however, your ears are affected by a change in pressure, and you might find yourself suffering from barotrauma, or pressure damage. To protect yourself,

As many as 85 percent of infections of the middle ear are experienced by children under 12.

0–5 YEARS

Help your child avoid infection

Breastfeeding offers some immunity to infections; in addition, the action of breastfeeding—a strong suck followed by a swallow—inhibits the flow of milk into the eustachian tube. Bottles, in contrast, can provoke infection because milk can pool and flow into the eustachian tube, where it provides a perfect breeding ground for bacteria. Some doctors believe that sucking a pacifier promotes the flow of fluids from a baby's mouth and into the eustachian tube and do not recommend it. Teaching children to blow their noses as early on as possible might prevent some episodes of ear infection by clearing mucus or fluid from the nasal cavity and preventing it from entering the middle ear.

- be alert to the risks of barotrauma when flying (see page 62),
- know the risks of any hobbies you enjoy, such as diving or bungee jumping, and
- take time to become acclimatized to altitude before exerting yourself. Nosebleeds, too, can be caused by a rapid change in air pressure and by exposure to high altitude.

TURN IT DOWN!

Sensorineural hearing loss—that caused by noise—is preventable. Your ears are not designed to listen to loud noise: If noise is loud enough and lasts long enough, it will damage your hearing. As exposure time increases, more and more nerve endings in the inner ear are destroyed, and they cannot regenerate. If you have grown used to a loud noise it has probably already damaged your ears, and no treatment will help (see page 80).

A GOOD NIGHT'S SLEEP

Unfortunately, you are not the only person who may be troubled by a problem with your ears, nose, or throat. Up to 25 percent of the population snores habitually, disturbing not only their own sleep, but also that of the people they live with. Snoring can be a serious social and medical problem.

Snoring occurs when the tongue and soft palate collapse during sleep, causing a blockage in the air passage, which prevents the sleeper from breathing normally. The sound produced is made by the collapsed parts of the mouth vibrating and striking each other during breathing. Snoring is most common in children and in people over 40 years old and can be the result of many factors, including swollen adenoids, alcohol, sleeping pills, being overweight, and smoking. You may also snore if your nose is blocked by a cold, hay fever, or nasal polyps.

Countless methods have been devised in an attempt to cure snoring, and they range from the age-old method of sewing a ball into the back of the pajamas to nasal sprays to headgear that repositions the jaw. It is true that such inventions are likely to stop you from snoring—but only by keeping you awake.

CHANGES FOR A SNORE-FREE NIGHT

Some simple lifestyle changes can have a great impact on your quality of sleep. None of the methods here need medical help, or require you to sleep in discomfort. Try them out and see which works for you, so that you and the people around you get a better night's sleep.

Be habitual *Establish regular sleeping patterns, and go to bed at the same time each night. Sleep deprivation can be a cause of snoring.*

Get fit *By getting more exercise and losing a few excess pounds, not only will you improve muscle tone, but you will also lose bulky neck tissue, which causes snoring by narrowing the airways.*

Eating and drinking *Don't eat for three hours before sleeping—saliva and mucus production can interfere with breathing—and don't drink alcohol for four hours because alcohol can overrelax the muscles. Drink a glass of warm milk before turning in, because milk contains an amino acid that induces sleep.*

Sleep naturally *Do not take sleeping pills or tranquilizers before going to bed; they relax the muscles too much.*

The right position *Go to sleep on your side rather than on your back, and prop your head up four inches with pillows.*

How your ENT change with age

As our bodies mature, the performance of our ears, nose, and throat changes. It generally deteriorates with age, but certain events in life, such as illness or pregnancy, can also have a profound effect on functioning.

HOW HEARING CHANGES

Periods of temporary hearing loss are common, particularly when associated with colds and other infections. Some degree of hearing loss, however, is a normal part of the aging process. Unfortunately, this is a permanent condition, but there are increasing numbers of aids that can be used to assist with hearing.

Age-related hearing loss

Permanent age-related hearing loss tends to occur in families. Referred to as presbycusis, this is usually associated with a genetic predisposition rather than noise trauma, although persistent exposure to loud noise also causes hearing loss (see page 80).

As hearing matures

At birth, our ears are sensitive to wavelengths between 40 and 20,000 Hz. A child can often distinguish sounds from 20 Hz (lowest note on an organ) to 20,000 Hz, and hearing stays within these frequencies in adulthood. As we age, it becomes less acute.

Generally, as age increases, so too does loss of hearing. It begins with loss of high-frequency sounds such as speech, particularly high-frequency consonants such as "t," "p," "k," and "f." Such hearing loss can often go undetected for quite some time because the onset is usually gradual: Most experts agree that it usually begins during our 50s, although some suggest it starts as early as the 30s.

The loss of the ability to both hear high-frequency sounds and to detect quiet sounds diminishes as we age. Some experts quantify hearing loss as mild, severe, and profound depending on a person's inability to distinguish sounds at particular levels. Mild hearing loss is the inability to hear 25–30 decibels—for example, above the background hum of a quiet office; severe loss is the inability to hear 40–60 decibels, the level of normal speech; and a person who cannot hear 90 decibels—for example, a loud radio—has profound hearing loss.

About a quarter of people 65–75 years old and half of those over 75 suffer from some degree of hearing loss. There are only 16,000 fine-hair sound detector cells in the average cochlea, and most people will have lost about one third of them by the time they are 65. These cells are irreplaceable.

Conductive hearing loss

It is not uncommon, either during childhood or adulthood, to experience a loss of hearing caused by a blockage that prevents sound from entering the inner ear. Such episodes of hearing loss are often temporary and can usually be treated easily, fully restoring hearing to normal. As we age, one of the more frequent reasons for this type of hearing loss is the buildup of ear wax. Ear wax becomes drier as we get older and is also more easily compacted. It is, however, a simple procedure to have it removed at the doctor's office (see pages 116–17).

Keeping tuned in

In so-called assistive listening devices, sound is amplified and delivered via headphones and earphones to enable you to hear a stereo, a telephone (either with an amplified handset or an extra earpiece), a television, or a radio.

Alarm calls

The usual sound signal in doorbells, alarm clocks, baby monitors, and smoke detectors can be changed to a flashing light or vibration system. Extensions or remote units can be situated in other rooms or simply moved around the house so that a light flashes when supper is ready, for example. Alarm clocks can be attached to vibration systems that wake you in bed.

DEVICES TO HELP WITH HEARING LOSS

Daily life is full of situations that can be frustrating for those with a degree of hearing loss and also those close to them: difficulty speaking on the telephone, for example, or having the television or radio turned up very loud.

Because many causes of adult hearing loss are untreatable, the major tasks of the doctor, audiologist, and hearing therapist are to prevent further hearing loss, if possible, and to rehabilitate remaining useful hearing. If you suspect that your hearing is not as acute as it once was, don't wait. The sooner you see a doctor, the better: Some aids take a little getting used to.

A wide range of equipment is available to aid hearing and communication, all of which may improve the quality of a person's life.

In your ear

There is a vast array of hearing aids suitable for most people with various causes of hearing loss. They act as an amplifier and improve the hearing that you have left: They cannot replace lost hearing. It can take weeks, if not months, to adjust to the amplified sounds, particularly for those who have been deaf for some time. Hearing aids can be worn on the body, behind the ear, and in the ear, and the most suitable type will depend on the cause and extent of an individual's hearing loss.

Staying in touch

A wide variety of state-of-the-art communication equipment is available. Devices such as text telephones and computerized notepads allow understanding of the spoken language, enable two-way communication without a human interpreter, improve reading skills, and help with learning sign languages.

Indoor environments

An induction loop fitted into a building converts sound signals into electrical impulses through a wire. The current sets up a magnetic field in the wire that can be picked up by a hearing aid switched to the correct setting. These sounds are unaffected by distance or background noise, so they are extremely useful in public places such as conference rooms, theaters, concert halls, ticket offices, and doctors' offices.

SCENTS IN THE RISE
A child's sense of smell matures from birth and is as acute as a young adult's by around the age of eight.

TESTING TIMES
Pregnancy is often a time of heightened sensitivity, with many stronger odors provoking nausea and vomiting.

THE DECLINE OF ADULTHOOD
The sense of smell certainly declines as we grow older, although the age at which this begins is debated.

THE CHANGING SENSE OF SMELL

Some people have a keener sense of smell than others, but we all experience a weakness or loss of smell—and often of the intertwined sense of taste with it—at some point during our lives.

For the most part, we tend to rely on our eyes and ears rather than our sense of smell to determine our social behavior. From an evolutionary point of view, this is an advanced state—dogs, for example, "follow their noses" for food, territory, finding family, and mating. Ants follow a complex system of social behavior patterns related to their sense of smell. Yet, mothers can recognize their own babies from smell alone in the same way that a newborn infant locates its mother's nipple by smell. Our ways of finding mates are also partially dependent on invisible smell signals from pheromones (see page 42).

A heightened sense of smell

Some people develop aversions to certain smells. This is by far most common in pregnancy and is closely connected to the nausea and vomiting of early pregnancy. During this time, the placenta produces increasing amounts of estrogen to keep the fetus healthy. A side effect of this is that women can detect volatile chemicals in, for example, coffee, tea, tobacco, petroleum products, perfume, and some foods, and find them intolerably strong. Pregnant women often say that it is a smell that triggers vomiting. It also seems that women who are born infertile, if helped to conceive, are less likely to suffer from morning

sickness. Research is ongoing to prove the exact links between estrogen and the sense of smell.

The taste–smell connection

Your senses of smell and taste are very closely linked. Both depend on the recognition of chemical molecules from substances around you, which stimulate specialized nerve cells in your nose, mouth, and throat. These nerve cells produce electrical impulses, which are taken to parts of the brain where smells and tastes are recognized. As many as 10,000 taste buds are located on the upper surface of your tongue, but these can only distinguish among sweet, sour, bitter, and salt stimuli. Other factors such as texture and temperature play a part in recognizing a particular "taste," but more important are the smell receptors high in the nasal cavity. Some flavors rely more on smell than taste for their identification. These include chocolate and coffee: If you hold your nose while you eat chocolate, all you will be able to tell is whether it is sweet or bitter.

A weakened sense of smell

Your sense of smell declines in old age. This is in keeping with the general loss of brain function that occurs with aging. The olfactory bulb—which carries smell from the odor detectors in the nasal cavity to the brain—gets smaller as we age and the nerve cells in the nose that detect smells become thinner and more spread out and so are less effective. This can be dangerous

Up to 1 in 10 people complain of problems with taste and smell at some time in their lives.

because it may lead to a reduced ability to detect dangerous smells such as gas or food that has gone bad.

A few people are born with a poor sense of smell, but the problem is usually an acquired one. You may lose your sense of smell temporarily if you have a stuffy nose, for example, or permanently after a serious head injury. Localized nasal problems, such as polyps or a deviated nasal septum, can also cause a loss of the sense of smell. Allergies can thicken the membrane lining the nose and thereby reduce smell acuity. Recent research has pointed to the loss of the sense of smell being an early sign of Alzheimer's disease, a condition that affects more women than men (see page 110). There have also been reported instances of temporary desensitization to smells. Workers in chocolate factories, for example, are

DO WOMEN HAVE A KEENER SENSE OF SMELL?

Women have a more sensitive and wider ranging sense of smell than men or children. This is thought to be because estrogen, the female hormone, increases the action of the olfactory nerve cells. Women are generally much more sensitive to the odor of musk, similar to the male hormone testosterone, than men, who are relatively insensitive. The level of a woman's sensitivity to this smell varies according to the stage in her menstrual cycle, again probably related to the amount of estrogen circulating. Women on the pill (who do not ovulate), women whose ovaries have been removed, and postmenopausal women have a less acute sense of smell and in some cases complain that they have completely lost their sense of smell.

reputed not to smell the chocolate after a while. However, the chocolate smells as strong to someone returning after a week's vacation as it does to a newcomer to the factory.

Professional noses

Although some people do have a better sense of smell than others, most who consider themselves good "noses" agree that this is primarily a matter of being aware of smells and of practice in noticing the distinctions between them.

49

YOUR CHANGING VOICE

From the high-pitched cry of a newborn baby to the deep bass tones of the adult man, our voices change as we age. Although these changes are most dramatic in adolescent males, all of our voices evolve at almost every stage of life.

Factors that influence our voices as we age include growth, which affects vocal cord length; the development of muscles in the neck; the changing structure of the tissues of the vocal cords; and the increasing boniness of cartilage of the larynx.

A child's voice

At birth, the vocal cords, which vibrate to produce sound, are about 0.79 inch long. Throughout childhood these grow about 0.03 inch each year in boys and 0.02 inch a year in girls. In spite of their smaller vocal cords and smaller lungs, however, children can produce sounds as loud as adults because they make sounds of a higher frequency. They also have a higher lung pressure that allows them to work harder than adults to produce sound.

> ## Human speech frequencies vary between 50 and 4000 Hz.

Changes at adolescence

Men and women have different voice pitches and this is directly related to the size of the larynx.

Testosterone production in boys from puberty onward causes their larynxes to lengthen, and thickens the vocal cords. This produces different pitches and harmonics. Initially, boys may alternate between their prepubertal high-pitched voices and deeper tones, sometimes producing a mix of the two as the boy becomes accustomed to the change, but gradually the deeper voice stabilizes.

The changes in girls' voices are less dramatic, but they do become increasingly breathless, husky, and lower in frequency.

Adulthood

The loudness and quality of your voice generally stabilize during the midlife years. However, the larynx slowly descends and thickens with age. A man's voice continues to deepen as he grows older, though after about age 70, its pitch goes up again slightly because of falling testosterone levels, and it can sound thinner and more reedy. A woman's voice, by contrast, becomes deeper and more husky. By the time men and women reach their 90s, they sound much the same; also, older people may speak more slowly, and their voices can sound more tremulous.

Combining voices
Voice pitch varies from male to female and with age. A successful singing ensemble exploits these differences.

What is a voiceprint?

Some experts argue that we each have an individual "voiceprint." Every person's vocal cords process sounds slightly differently, and the way each person produces sound—the use of the tongue, mouth, lips, and so on—also differs. The combination of these factors makes it unlikely that two voices would be exactly alike. The voiceprint is a tracing measured on a machine called a spectrograph registering how high and low a voice is and its Hz frequency. Although critics argue against the accuracy of voiceprints, they have been used in criminal investigations.

ASK THE EXPERT

Looking out for symptoms

You will experience symptoms from your ears, nose, and throat fairly frequently. As with other body systems, the important thing is knowing how to distinguish between what is serious and what is trivial.

Recognizing the various symptoms that can indicate an ear, nose, or throat problem will help you to decide on your best course of action. If you are not sure whether your symptoms require a visit to the doctor, call the nurse practitioner for advice. Persistent symptoms, even if they appear trivial, should prompt a visit to the doctor.

NOSEBLEEDS
A nosebleed in a child with a cold is not usually cause for concern, although the nasal lining may be likely to bleed again if the nose is blown too enthusiastically. Encourage frequent light nose blowing (see page 44). Nosebleeds at other times may run in the family and are usually no cause for concern: Children grow out of them by their teens. However, consult a doctor if a child with a nosebleed
• is pale, sweaty, and unresponsive;
• has lost a lot of blood;
• has had a blow to the nose; or
• is vomiting blood.
Nosebleeds in adults can be an indication of something more serious such as high blood pressure. A nosebleed that doesn't stop after 15 minutes is a medical emergency.

SINUS PAIN
Sometimes it is difficult to distinguish between an ordinary headache and one caused by blocked or infected sinuses. If the answer to any of the following questions is yes, the pain may be caused by sinus disease and you should see your doctor.

• Do you feel the pain mainly in your face and forehead?
• Does the pain worsen when you bend over?
• Have you recently had a runny nose and high temperature?
• Do you have a discolored or blood-stained nasal discharge?

EARACHES
Earaches are much more common in young children. If your baby or toddler is screaming and pulling his or her ears, suspect a middle ear infection (acute otitis media). These symptoms may also be associated with a discharge of pus, and sometimes blood, if the eardrum has perforated. Your child should see a doctor, who will prescribe antibiotics.

In adults, too, earaches may signify a middle ear infection. If it is accompanied by a blocked sensation in the ear, it may be due to pressure damage or eustachian tube malfunction. Pain that is worse if you pull on your outer ear may be caused by a boil in the ear canal or possibly an infection of the skin of the ear canal (acute otitis externa).

Discharge from the ear
In children and adults, this is commonly associated with an infection of the outer ear canal, which might also accompany a sore, itchy, and painful ear, or a perforated eardrum. Causes may include swimmer's ear, eczema, psoriasis, or (especially in children) a foreign body in the ear.

Hold your nose
A person with a nosebleed should sit with his or her head upright and pinch both nostrils together for at least 15 minutes. The method of tipping the head back simply allows blood to trickle down the throat, causing coughing.

Middle ear infection
An infection may also cause discharge if the eardrum develops a hole so that pus and blood escape. This usually relieves the severe pain. A clear or blood-stained discharge from the ear or nose after an injury needs emergency medical treatment.

COLDS
At least 200 viruses are known to cause the common cold, and you are more likely to succumb in fall or

ASSESSING LOSS OF HEARING

If you have any concerns about your ability to hear, ask yourself these questions to decide whether to see the doctor.

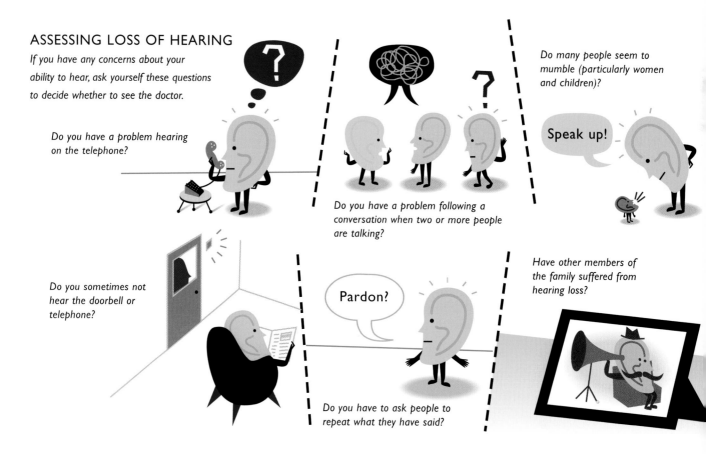

Do you have a problem hearing on the telephone?

Do you have a problem following a conversation when two or more people are talking?

Do many people seem to mumble (particularly women and children)?

Speak up!

Do you sometimes not hear the doorbell or telephone?

Pardon?

Have other members of the family suffered from hearing loss?

Do you have to ask people to repeat what they have said?

winter. The symptoms of sneezing, stuffy or runny nose, sore throat, and fever develop between 12 hours and 3 days after catching the infection. Colds are minor self-limiting illnesses lasting only a few days, unless you develop complications, which are more likely in children and older people. Children commonly develop ear infections after a cold; adults may have sinusitis or a chest infection.

Stuffy or runny nose
The membrane lining your nose can swell and produce fluid for a number of reasons. The most common by far is a virus infection, or common cold. A blocked nose may also be caused by an anatomical distortion of the nose by nasal polyps or after a fracture. If you are also suffering an itchy nose and eyes,

then the likely cause is allergy. If the symptoms are seasonal, this may be an allergy to pollen, molds, or spores and is called seasonal rhinitis; if it is persistent, it is likely to be caused by dust mites.

Sneezing
This is the nose's defense mechanism to try to expel unwanted substances. It can be caused by an allergy, irritant, or infection.

SORE THROAT
Soreness in the throat may be caused by exposure to either pollutants or irritants such as cigarette smoke. In addition, shouting and other voice stressors can cause a sore throat (see page 68).

Soreness of the throat along with a fever and aches and pains may indicate tonsillitis. Sore throat, fever,

and swollen glands in your neck, armpits, or groin could indicate glandular fever. You should visit the doctor in both cases.

IT'S NOT TRUE!

"Nasal discharge tells you what's wrong"

Some people believe that clear nasal discharge indicates a viral infection, and yellow-green discharge means a bacterial infection. The color of the discharge, however, simply reflects the number of white blood cells fighting off the infection. A yellowish discharge means that white blood cell production is in full swing.

Do people complain that you turn the television up too loud?

Have you worked in a noisy environment?

Some prescription drugs such as certain antibiotics can cause a drop in the white blood cell count, which may provoke a sore throat.

Hoarseness, loss of voice

Hoarseness is a change in quality or volume of your voice caused by alteration in your vocal cords, which can swell or develop nodules from overuse. This can be due to a viral infection (the common cold or laryngitis), specific occupations such as singing or teaching, or pollutants and irritants such as cigarette smoke.

If your voice has changed slowly at the same time as your skin and hair have become dry or you feel excessively tired, you may have an underactive thyroid gland. In smokers, a hoarse voice can be a symptom of a more serious problem such as throat or lung cancer.

Difficulty swallowing

If accompanied by a sore throat, a swallowing problem may be caused by an object lodged in your throat. If you feel that food gets stuck in your throat, or if you feel a lump in your throat, you may have acid reflux. This can also cause a recurrent cough and a sore throat. Anxiety can cause the sensation of a lump in the throat, but in such cases swallowing is normal.

HEARING PROBLEMS

Up to 1 in 1,000 newborn babies is profoundly deaf and nearly 1 in 20 has significant hearing impairment. Screening tests are available, and babies benefit from early intervention. Tell your doctor if you suspect a hearing deficiency from your baby's reactions to noise.

Problems in older children can be harder to pinpoint because some children seem to "screen out" adults deliberately, but a child who needs the television turned up louder than normal should probably be checked. Hearing problems can also cause underperformance at school, so if your child's performance seems to have worsened, suspect hearing difficulties. Possible causes for this are inherited forms of deafness, an infection such as rubella, or middle ear infection.

In adults, hearing loss can affect all sounds or just some frequencies, and it may be sudden or gradual. There may be a family history of deafness. Other possibilities are overexposure to loud noise or wax buildup in the outer ear canal. Half of all people over 70 have some degree of age-related hearing loss, and people should discuss coping strategies with their doctor and family sooner rather than later (see page 47).

Does milk cause mucus production?

TALKING POINT

Despite many scientific studies on the subject, contrary medical opinions, and anecdotal evidence, there has been no scientific evidence to link mucus production with milk. Many people find that drinking milk leaves a soft filmy coating in the mouth and throat, but this substance should not be confused with mucus. A recent study in Australia found that the "mucus effect" of cow's milk is most likely just the milk itself, probably combined with slightly increased saliva levels, and not an increase in mucus production. An inability to tolerate milk products is likely to be lactose intolerance, or in rare cases, milk allergy.

Sudden hearing loss in one ear only is an emergency because it can result in permanent hearing loss; seek urgent medical help. The most common cause for this is a viral infection, but occasionally a benign tumor on the auditory nerve is diagnosed.

Tinnitus

Tinnitus sufferers hear persistent noises in the ear, indicating damage to the middle or inner ear. The noises may be high or low in pitch, they may be buzzing or sibilant, and they can continue night and day. Possible causes include Meniere's disease, exposure to loud noise, and certain medication, such as aspirin, taken in high doses, but in many cases there is no identifiable cause.

How infections are spread

Infections of the ears, nose, and throat are common, partly because these organs are the main entrance to the body through which all food, fluid, and air pass. As such, they offer free entry to a host of bacteria and viruses, too.

Infectious diseases are caused by microorganisms that invade your body. They cause inflammation and immune responses that then produce symptoms of a particular illness.

VIRUSES

Most ear, nose, and throat infections are caused by viruses, some others by bacteria, and relatively few by fungi or parasites. Viruses can only grow or divide in living cells. More than 200 different viruses can cause the common cold.

Airborne disease

Viruses pass from person to person in droplets of mucus produced by an already infected person. The virus particles are expelled by coughing or sneezing and inhaled, affecting the mucous membrane of the recipient. Even when a tissue is used, the droplet range for a sneeze can be several feet. One study found that in the infectious stage of a cold more than 6,000 viable droplets were produced every hour, and these can remain airborne for up to 10 minutes.

Contact contamination

Cold viruses can also live for some hours on skin and other surfaces, so picking up a child, handing someone a plate or the TV remote control, or sharing a towel can all spread the infection, as can shaking a contaminated hand. If you have a cold, be sure to wash your hands often to avoid spreading it to others.

WHO GETS INFECTIONS?

It is also important to remember that an individual's chances of catching a cold depend on several factors:
- The length of exposure: 8 hours a day in close contact with an infected person increases the risk.
- Health status: Someone whose immunity is compromised is more likely to catch a cold, so the old and young are especially at risk.

A CHILD'S ENVIRONMENT CHILDREN ARE PARTICULARLY VULNERABLE TO INFECTIONS. EVERY DAY THAT KATE COMES INTO CONTACT WITH THE OTHER CHILDREN AT HER SCHOOL, THERE IS THE CHANCE SHE MIGHT PICK UP A COLD OR OTHER INFECTION.

9:15 KATE'S MOTHER, WHO IS A NURSE, IS NOT OVERLY CONCERNED. ALTHOUGH NO ONE LIKES BEING SICK, EACH ILLNESS HELPS BUILD KATE'S IMMUNE SYSTEM. SHE HAS NO QUALMS ABOUT KATE ATTENDING SCHOOL.

3:30 MANY CHILDREN OF THIS AGE HAVE NOT ACQUIRED IMMUNITY TO A NUMBER OF THE MOST COMMON DISEASES YET, AND KATE IS NO EXCEPTION. BY THE END OF THE DAY SHE HAS A SORE THROAT AND HER NOSE IS BECOMING STUFFY.

12:45 AIRBORNE VIRUSES ARE HARD TO AVOID WHEN CHILDREN SNEEZE AND COUGH. DISEASES CAN ALSO BE PASSED BY CONTACT CONTAMINATION, SUCH AS WHEN KATE SHARES A DRINK WITH A COLD-RIDDEN FRIEND.

THE NEXT DAY BY KEEPING KATE AT HOME, HER MOTHER CAN MAKE SURE KATE GETS REST AND PLENTY OF FLUIDS AND SEES THE DOCTOR IF HER CONDITION GETS WORSE. SHE KNOWS THAT KATE IS INFECTIOUS AND DECIDES TO KEEP HER AWAY FROM HER BROTHERS, WHO MIGHT CATCH THE BUG.

Self-help for ENT problems

Illnesses of the ENT are some of the most common, and treatment is widely and readily available. Understanding the advantages and disadvantages of different treatments helps you to choose the most appropriate remedy.

OVER-THE-COUNTER DRUGS

Many medications intended for treating ear, nose, and throat illnesses are available over the counter without a doctor's prescription. Keep in mind that even drugs available over the counter can have side effects or may not be suitable for you. Always read the information on the package or ask the pharmacist for advice.

Your medicine cabinet

A number of over-the-counter drugs can effectively combat common symptoms. However, those for illness of the ears, nose, and throat often contain more than you bargained for, and you should be aware of pitfalls with these generally useful drugs.

Painkillers

Effective painkillers for treating headaches, sore throats, fevers, and general cold and flu symptoms include acetaminophen, ibuprofen, and aspirin. However, all can be dangerous if taken inappropriately.

Aspirin should not be given to children under 12 years old or taken if you are breastfeeding. It can cause gastric irritation and even ulceration. Those allergic to aspirin may develop life-threatening anaphylaxis and should carefully check the labels of cold remedies to avoid aspirin.

Acetaminophen is extremely dangerous if the maximum safe and recommended dosage is exceeded— as few as 20 tablets taken in a 24-hour period can cause severe liver damage in an adult and, less frequently, acute kidney failure. If you suspect acetaminophen overdose, seek urgent medical help.

Ibuprofen can cause gastric irritation and, in theory, can worsen asthma. Those allergic to aspirin should not take ibuprofen or similar drugs, and neither should these drugs be taken during pregnancy or while breastfeeding. If you suffer from high blood pressure, consult your doctor before starting the drug.

Cough remedies

A wide variety of cough remedies is available over the counter, mainly containing various drugs in a flavored syrup base. The effectiveness of cough remedies is doubtful, which is why they are rarely prescribed by doctors, and there is no hard evidence that expectorants—medicines that encourage sputum production in order to make it easier to cough up—are effective at all. Suppressants, which suppress the cough reflex, may be helpful at night because they contain codeine and similar drugs that may help you get a good night's rest. However, these drugs can cause constipation. Also, codeine can be habit-forming and for this reason, many pharmacists prefer it to be prescribed by a doctor.

positive health tips

Using over-the-counter medicines wisely

Before you take any medication, whether prescribed or purchased, you should always check the following:

- What is the correct dosage?

- Is the drug still good? Many drugs have an expiration date printed somewhere in the packaging after which they may lose their efficacy or, in some cases, be dangerous to take.

- Are there instructions about when to take the drug (such as before or after food, or at bedtime)?

- Make sure you do not take different drugs with the same ingredients that could result in accidental overdose, or that do not interact well. If in doubt, consult the pharmacist.

- How long is it safe to take a drug before seeking advice from a health professional? This should be printed on the package.

- Keep medicines in a lockable cabinet out of reach of children, and check the contents regularly to dispose of out-of-date drugs.

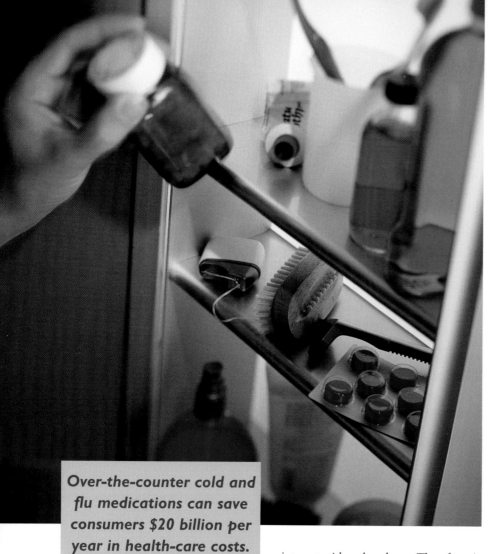

Over-the-counter cold and flu medications can save consumers $20 billion per year in health-care costs.

Antihistamines

These are often contained in cold and flu remedies because they dry up mucus production. They are also useful in treating allergic conditions such as hay fever. Side effects include drowsiness, but this varies depending on which kind you take.

Decongestants

These help to alleviate a blocked or runny nose and are available in tablet and capsule form, and as sprays and drops. They cease to be effective after a week, however, after which they can cause worsening of the original symptoms. Topical decongestant drugs can affect your heart rate and raise your blood pressure if absorbed in great enough quantities, and they can interact with other drugs. Therefore, it is wise to avoid using them if possible.

Cold and flu remedies

There are many medicines available over the counter, so it is worth talking to a pharmacist about their potential benefits and disadvantages. Some contain unhelpful ingredients, such as caffeine; others can be dangerous if they interact with other drugs. Some people have become addicted to these compound remedies. Dosage instructions can be complicated and overdoses are dangerous. Generally, it's easier to stick to individual drugs.

Eardrops

Various drops are available over the counter. Some of these can make the skin sore after a few days' use and others are available to soothe irritated skin, but are not effective for earaches. They never cure earaches—you need to see a doctor to determine the cause.

Sore throat remedies

These are available as lozenges to suck and sprays for the throat. Most preparations available for sore throats contain mixtures of antiseptic, flavorings, and painkillers. Some sprays contain local anesthetics, which not only deaden pain sensation but also perception of hot and cold—be careful not to burn your throat after using a spray.

MEDICINE FOR CHILDREN

Children can be far more sensitive to drugs than adults, so it is vital when administering drugs to children to read the labels carefully to find out dosage, delivery, and timing and to follow the directions exactly. If you are at all unsure of any of the directions, contact your pharmacist. Only combine medications with your doctor's advice.

Use your pharmacist wisely

Cut down on unnecessary visits to the doctor by consulting a pharmacist first. A pharmacist will be able to give advice on:

- *Whether your symptoms are the result of a potentially serious condition or not.*
- *Whether another medication you are taking rules out a particular over-the-counter remedy.*
- *If a remedy is suitable if you are pregnant or breastfeeding.*

COMPLEMENTARY THERAPIES

Recent years have seen a boom in the demand for complementary therapy (alternative medicine used with traditional treatment) as an increasing number of people develop resistance to antibiotics and turn to alternative methods for solutions to their medical problems.

Many schools of alternative medicine have roots in ancient tradition; all place an emphasis on the health and well-being of the whole body as the basis for curing or alleviating specific ailments. Fundamental to alternative medicine is an awareness of what constitutes a healthy diet and how what you eat may determine the optimal functioning of your immune system, which is vital in maintaining the health of your ears, nose, and throat (see page 64). In some cases, this may result in the elimination of entire food groups from the diet in order to alleviate or cure symptoms.

Homeopathy

First developed in the late 18th century, homeopathy aims to enhance the body's natural tendency to heal itself. Patients are treated with minute doses of a plant, animal, or mineral substance that would cause the same symptoms in a healthy person if taken in excess. In other words, homeopathy is the practice of treating like with like. Usually administered in pill form, treatments are so diluted as to be harmless to babies, children, and during pregnancy. Homeopathy is a precise science with many remedies to treat most conditions, depending on what the specific symptoms are.

Aromatherapy

Treatment using scents can be traced back to the worlds of ancient Egypt and Greece. It involves the use of oils extracted from plants, flowers, seeds, barks, roots, and leaves to provide physical and psychological therapeutic relief for a wide range of ailments.

All essential oils have natural healing properties that, once absorbed into the body either by inhalation or through the skin, display antiseptic qualities. Some act as antidepressants, some as pain relievers, and others are antiviral or antiinflammatory. The attraction of such treatment is that the oils

Don't go it alone

Complementary therapies are not intended as a replacement for orthodox treatments but should rather work with them in order to provide relief—hence the term complementary. You should always consult your doctor before taking any course of action and should not rely on self-diagnosis. Complementary treatment is almost always tailored to suit an individual's needs, with the result that remedies for similar ailments may vary from person to person.

have a positive effect on the whole body—both mentally and physically —and without side effects if used properly. Different oils can be effective for different problems of the ears, nose, and throat (see page 58). Add two to three drops of the appropriate oil to a tissue, place near your nose (not touching), and inhale. Or prepare a steam inhalation by adding five to seven drops of an oil to a bowl of just-boiled water. Hold

Homeopathic remedies for ear problems

SYMPTOMS	TREATMENT
Pain in the ears when babies are teething	Chamomile 30 Every 2 hours for 1 day
Acute pain with discharge from the nose and ears	Mercuris solubillis 30 Every 2 hours for 2–3 days
Pain in the ears without deafness or discharge	Mullein oil 3–4 drops in the ear 2–3 times a day for 1 day
Pain with discharge from the ears	Pulsatilla 30 (right) Every 4 hours for 2 days

your face over the bowl and breathe deeply and rhythmically for several minutes. To intensify the effect, shroud your head and the bowl with a towel to trap the steam.

Western herbalism

Like aromatherapy, herbalism exploits the natural healing properties of plants, but herbal remedies are taken in a variety of forms, including tinctures, tablets, teas, compresses, and also in their natural state. They can be used to alleviate many symptoms or to prevent illness from developing in the first place. Chewing on ginger, for example, can alleviate or prevent travel sickness (see page 60).

Auricular therapy

Whereas the most common complementary therapies concentrate on alleviating and curing coughs, colds, and fevers, there is one school that focuses on the ears—auricular therapy. A branch of acupuncture, it works on the theory that there are about 300 points on energy channels on the ear, each of which represents a different part of the human body,

and that any given pain can be alleviated by applying pressure—using either fingers or an acupunture needle, or sometimes a laser or magnet—to the corresponding point on the ear. Although auricular therapy deals for the most part with the body as a whole, some success has been reported in the relief and treatment of sinus problems and tinnitus.

Ten essential oils for ears, nose, and throat

All of these oils except garlic may be added to a steam inhalation, which provides instant and lasting relief. Several may be gargled.* Garlic oil is applied as eardrops.

SYMPTOM OR CONDITION	ESSENTIAL OIL
Sinusitis, fever, nausea, vertigo	Peppermint
Common cold, flu	Lemon
Common cold, cough, fever, flu, sinusitis	Eucalyptus
Common cold, flu, sinusitis, whooping cough	Tea tree
Common cold, flu, laryngitis, sore throat	Thyme*
Earaches, whooping cough, vertigo	Lavender*
Cough, sore throat	Hyssop*
Earaches	Garlic
Throat infections, sore throat, laryngitis, tonsillitis	Clary sage*
Earaches, nausea	Chamomile

The auricular map
Auricular therapists believe that the ear is a map of an inverted body. Points representing the head and neck are generally located on or near the lobe, and those representing the feet are at the top of the external ear.

Different types of acupuncture
Auricular acupuncture differs from regular acupuncture because it works on pressure points to tap directly into the central nervous system, rather than opening the energy channels to release the flow of "chi" or energy throughout the body.

Esophagus

Throat

Throat

Back of neck

Lower jaw

Teeth

Eyes

Face

Trouble-free traveling

Motion sickness is common but by no means inevitable. There are several tried-and-true drugs as well as many commonsense precautions you can take to reduce your risk of suffering.

Also known as travel sickness or *mal de mer*, motion sickness is a common problem in childhood that tends to be less of a nuisance as you get older. However, in severe rough waters, whole shiploads of people can be affected.

Research suggests that some people are seasick because they expect to be; conquering this feeling can keep you well.

WHAT CAUSES MOTION SICKNESS?

The symptoms are brought on when the brain receives conflicting messages from the sensory input of the eyes, the balance organs, and the body's spatial receptors. For example, if you are traveling by car and reading at the same time, your eyes send the message to your brain that you are stationary, whereas your inner ear tells the brain that you are moving. This sets off a chain of self-perpetuating reactions in the unconscious part of the brain.

WHAT ARE THE SYMPTOMS?

The symptoms at their mildest include a feeling of discomfort and uneasiness. As things get worse, you can start to feel sick and then develop a headache, dizziness, and fatigue. If the motion continues you can feel worse still, with sweating, pallor, yawning, and hyperventilation all occurring. Vomiting is common and can be prolonged and severe.

Recent research has reported that a large number of U.S. space shuttle astronauts suffer from motion sickness, particularly in the first two or three days of their mission. This is largely because of the repeated sudden head movements. Emotional factors and anxiety are also likely to be involved.

Research has been carried out on the effects of ginger root in combating "space sickness," but biofeedback techniques seem to have the greatest effect on reducing motion sickness in space. Through these techniques, astronauts are taught to take control of bodily functions that are generally considered to be involuntary, such as monitoring breathing and heart rate.

BEATING TRAVEL SICKNESS

Being tired makes your body less able to cope with motion sickness, so try to get a good night's sleep before you travel.

Spinning around
Many astronauts experience "space sickness," a condition that scientists believe is similar to the motion sickness we feel here on earth.

MOTION SICKNESS

Women are four times as likely as men to be seasick. Researchers have measured the stomach activity of men and women subjected to movements similar to those that induce motion sickness and, although they found comparable activity, the women were far more likely to say they felt sick. Research on round-the-world yachtswomen has shown that nausea is closely linked to the menstrual cycle and is usually worse in the three days before and first few days of a menstrual period, prompting theories that it may be linked to hormone levels.

Ginger: the travel drug?
There is some evidence that ginger— as tea, ale, or crystallized candy —has a beneficial effect on motion sickness. It is believed to act on the gastrointestinal system rather than on the balance mechanism.

Drugs

Drugs for travel sickness must be taken in advance.

You can buy some over the counter, whereas others are only available with a doctor's prescription. Some may cause drowsiness, and you should note the risk of driving after taking these drugs. Some also interact with alcohol and other drugs affecting the brain. Scopolamine is the most effective and is available by prescription as a patch. It should not be taken if you have glaucoma, and it can cause drowsiness, vision problems, and a dry mouth, although this is not usually a problem at the small doses involved. Stick the patch onto your skin 5–6 hours before your trip. The effect lasts up to 72 hours, which is particularly useful on board ship. Bonine is an over-the-counter alternative, but it is not available in patch form. Antihistamine drugs also have an effect on motion sickness and are available for adults and children. Dramamine is available over the counter.

Pressure wristbands

If you are wary of potential side effects of drugs, you could try elastic acupressure wristbands. One is worn on each wrist, like a watch or sweatband, and incorporates a button attached to the inner side. This applies constant pressure to the P6 meridian point on each wrist and can considerably lessen the effects of motion sickness. Compared to most drugs, there are no side effects and the benefits are immediate—you simply put them on 5–10 minutes before you set off.

Break up your trip

If it is possible, having a break in your trip can help your system to adjust and lessen feelings of motion sickness. This may add an hour to your journey but will be worth the delay.

Have a meal or snack

In some cases, the fear of travel sickness puts a person off eating before traveling, which makes the situation worse. A light meal helps to settle the stomach before a journey and reduces the likelihood of motion sickness. Try to eat a small meal before setting out, but avoid spicy or fatty foods. Eating plain cookies or crackers or sucking on mints during the journey can also help.

Stay hydrated

Take frequent sips of water during the trip and, if you are sick, be sure to replace the fluids you have lost. Avoid alcohol and caffeine.

CHOOSE YOUR SEAT WISELY

Where you sit can help prevent or alleviate motion sickness. Always travel where your eyes will see the same motion that your inner ears and body will experience, to prevent conflicting messages being sent to the brain. So, for example, in a car, sit in the front and look forward. Do not attempt to read: Even map reading can provoke feelings of sickness.

If possible, consider your environment before you travel: If you are going on a cruise and are prone to seasickness, choose your season of travel and geographical location with care. Try to avoid destinations where there are likely to be rough seas, and make sure you will have the opportunity to sit out on deck.

Flying high
If you tend to feel nauseated, try to choose a seat over the wing and sit by a window so that you can see the direction of travel. If the wing seats are gone, sit as close to the middle of the plane as you can.

On board ship
To avoid seasickness, don't lie in your cabin, but go on deck so that you can see the horizon. Bigger is definitely better when it comes to ships, and those with stabilizers are better still.

Train travel
Those sensitive to motion sickness may find train travel to be a problem, particularly on fast trains. If this applies to you, reserve a window seat facing the direction of travel and look out the window.

EARS AND AIR PRESSURE

Ear problems related to a change in environmental air pressure are very common and can result in temporary pain and hearing loss.

When ears pop

The middle ear normally contains air at atmospheric pressure. Usually, when you swallow, air enters your middle ear from your mouth via the eustachian tube and is absorbed by the membrane lining the middle ear. In this way, the pressure stays constant. If the eustachian tube is blocked for any reason, the middle ear pressure drops, pulling the eardrum inward, stretching it, and causing pain. If it remains blocked, the middle ear starts to fill with fluid produced from the membrane lining the middle ear.

Air travel

When you travel by air your middle ear is exposed to rapid changes in air pressure and so you must swallow frequently to equalize the middle ear pressure—it pays to stay awake during takeoff and landing in order to ensure this happens. Equalizing the pressure cannot happen properly if your eustachian tubes are blocked, however, and if this happens you can experience discomfort.

Be alert

Maintaining constant pressure is also important in other situations when you change altitude rapidly, such as during a deep-sea dive. Pilots and divers are taught to equalize pressure by practicing regular controlled swallowing and other tricks devised to ensure that the eustachian tubes are kept open.

The Valsalva maneuver

If the natural methods on the right do not work, you can try the Valsalva maneuver. You may already be accustomed to doing this without realizing that the technique had an official name.

1. Hold your nostrils closed.
2. Breathe in and close your mouth.
3. Force air backward into the back of your nose using your cheek and throat muscles.

If this is successful, you will hear a pop and feel the pressure change in your middle ear. The maneuver can be repeated as often as necessary.

Natural ear "poppers"
The different techniques used to equalize middle ear pressure vary only slightly; they all use the same method of opening the eustachian tube.

Yawn or simply open your mouth wide as if to yawn.

Feed your baby or give her a pacifier to suck.

Suck on a piece of candy or chew gum on takeoff and landing.

HEALTHY LIVING FOR YOUR ENT

Lifestyle factors exert a great influence over the health of the whole body, including the ears, nose, and throat. Every day we make choices that influence their health, including whether to smoke, what we eat, how much and what type of exercise we get, and whether we overstress our voices.

Foods for healthy ENT

The health of the ears, nose, and throat is dependent on a balanced diet with an emphasis on a few specific vitamins and nutrients that help to boost our ability to fight off infections and pollutants.

The close link among the ears, nose, and throat means that, once one area suffers from an infection, the others may well follow. Although there aren't any specific foods to boost the health of individual organs within the ENT system, a balanced diet plays an important role in maintaining their overall health—in particular, a diet that focuses on maintaining optimum health of the immune system.

KEEPING THE BALANCE

The simplest way to maintain a balanced diet is to remember the recommended ratios to one another of the five different groups that make up the foods we eat. The first group includes bread, cereals, and potatoes, providers of carbohydrates and fiber, and should form the basis of your diet, with 6 to 11 servings a day. Fruit and vegetables, excellent sources of vitamin C, carotenes, folates, and fiber, make up the next group, from which you should aim to eat at least five servings a day. Balance this with two servings of milk and dairy foods —for calcium, protein, and vitamins B_{12}, A, and D—and two servings of meat, legumes, fish, or tofu, for protein, iron, the B vitamins, zinc, and magnesium. Finally, include only a sparing number of foods that contain fat and sugar. Once this basic diet is established, you will be able to concentrate on the foods that contribute specifically to the health of your ears, nose, and throat.

MAINTAINING A HEALTHY MUCOUS MEMBRANE

Any airborne irritant that escapes the automatic filtering of the nose encounters the mucous membrane that lines the passages of the nose and throat. Keeping this membrane healthy is vital for fighting infections.

Vitamin B_2

Vitamin B_2, or riboflavin, contributes to the health of the mucous membrane. Rich sources include liver, milk, cheese, yogurt, eggs, green vegetables, yeast extract, and fortified breakfast cereals. A viscous substance produced by the mucous membrane traps foreign bacteria and destroys it using a chemical called lysozyme. A deficiency of vitamin B_2 causes a change to the mucous membrane, and this process may slow down, thus weakening the strength of the nose's defense against bacteria, and exposing the body to a greater risk of infection to the epiglottis, tonsils, pharynx, or larynx.

Vitamin A

An important vitamin for optimum functioning of the mucous membrane, vitamin A can be found in two forms: as retinol in foods from animals and as carotenoids in foods from plant sources. Animal sources of vitamin A include milk, fortified margarine, butter, cheese, egg yolk, liver, and fatty fish such as salmon, mackerel, and trout. Vegetable sources of vitamin A include carrots, tomatoes, and dark green vegetables.

ENT *SUPERFOODS*

All whole, unprocessed foods are good for the immune system, helping it fight off infections, but some foods are particularly effective at keeping your ears, nose, and throat in good health.

MUESLI Packed with B vitamins—including the all-important B_{12}—muesli and other whole-grain cereals mixed with nuts, seeds, and dried fruits, are good providers of minerals and vitamins.

SALMON Like many oily fish, salmon is a reliable source of the antioxidants vitamin E and selenium.

BLACK CURRANTS Amazingly, these tiny currants are one of the richest sources of vitamin C, with 4 oz. of fruit yielding approximately 0.0071 oz.

MANGO This is the best fruit source of antioxidant carotenoids and one of the very few fruit sources of vitamin E.

ONIONS Along with **GARLIC**, onions contain natural antibiotics, which are believed to bring relief from the symptoms of colds and the flu.

HEALTHFUL ANTIOXIDANTS

Although colds and the flu are spread rapidly from one person to the next, you are more likely to succumb if your immune system is weak. This leaves you with lower resistance for fighting infections. The key to optimum functioning of the immune system is a good intake of antioxidants, essential for "mopping up" free radicals. Antioxidants include vitamins C and E, carotenoids (plant sources of vitamin A), and the minerals selenium, zinc, and magnesium, which protect the body's cells from being damaged by free radicals. Zinc plays a particularly important role in the functioning of the immune system, and a deficiency is associated with a range of immunological defects, although they can be reversed once there is adequate zinc in the diet.

What are free radicals?

Free radicals are produced by the body's normal metabolic processes, and if they are allowed to build up they can cause damage to key components in the body such as DNA (the cell's building blocks), protein, and fat. Cells in which damage to the DNA is not repaired are more likely to develop cancer. Free radicals can also oxidize polyunsaturated fatty acids in foods and in cell membranes in the body to compounds called peroxides, which can damage cells. Antioxidants inhibit the oxidation of polyunsaturated fatty acids.

HELPING A COLD

Certain foods and drinks may help alleviate cold symptoms in the ears, nose, and throat and can offer a natural alternative to over-the-counter drugs.

Honey and lemon

It is likely that any warm drink will have a soothing effect on inflamed surfaces and thus provide relief from a sore throat and cough. A sweet and bitter hot drink, most commonly containing honey and lemon, is likely to be more tasty during a time when the sense of taste is affected. Honey has antiseptic and expectorant qualities that may also contribute to alleviating a sore throat, and lemon is rich in vitamin C.

Menthol

Menthol is a component of peppermint and eucalyptus oils and has been used over the centuries to provide relief from nasal congestion. Nowadays, menthol is commonly contained in cough lozenges and helps relieve the discomfort a cold can cause by imparting a cooling sensation that is felt in the nose and throat. The effect is temporary, rather like that of a localized anesthetic.

Garlic

Garlic contains compounds called ajoene, which may have antibacterial effects, and allicin, a powerful natural antibiotic. Both of these substances are thought to prevent the common cold and relieve troublesome symptoms.

According to the Common Cold Centre based at Cardiff University in Wales, spicy and hot foods, particularly those including ginger and chili, are decongestants, promoting airway secretions, which can have a calming effect on an inflamed throat.

A good week for antioxidants

It is not difficult to enjoy a delicious diet rich in antioxidants—they are readily available in many of the foods found in our supermarkets and convenience stores. The key is knowing which foods and how best to combine them to achieve a healthy and balanced diet. This week of menus should start you off with some ideas.

Some easy ways to increase the antioxidants in your diet include the following:

- Start the day with a bowl of whole-grain cereal and low-fat milk.
- Snack on nuts, dried fruits, or crispbread.
- Eat vegetable soup for lunch.
- Replace a cup of tea or coffee with a citrus fruit juice.
- Add a fresh salad to your evening meal.

positive health tips

The best sources of antioxidants

- Vitamin C: fresh fruit—especially citrus fruits and black currants, green vegetables, and potatoes

- Vitamin E: vegetable oils, nuts, vegetables, and cereals

- Carotenoids: carrots, tomatoes, and dark green vegetables

- Selenium: whole-grain cereals, meat, fish, cheese, and eggs

- Zinc: milk, cheese, meat, eggs, fish, whole-grain cereals, and legumes

- Magnesium: whole-grain cereals, nuts, and spinach

Day One
BREAKFAST
glass of orange juice
2 slices of whole-grain toast with black currant jelly
herbal tea
LUNCH
carrot and coriander soup
slice of whole-grain bread
natural yogurt
DINNER
grilled chicken breast with brown rice
tomato, mango, peppers, and onion salsa

Day Two
BREAKFAST
glass of grapefruit juice
muesli with extra sunflower seeds and low-fat milk
lemon tea
LUNCH
mayonnaise, spinach, and tomato sandwich with whole-grain bread
orange
DINNER
poached salmon, brown rice, and broccoli
green salad with nuts

Day Three
BREAKFAST
2 soft-boiled eggs
2 slices of whole-grain bread
lemon tea
LUNCH
tuna and corn sandwich with whole-grain bread
apple
DINNER
pork fillet kebab
spinach, onion, and chickpea salad
fruit salad

Day Four
BREAKFAST
glass of orange juice
bowl of bran cereal with handful of berries
LUNCH
crab and avocado salad
French bread
DINNER
lentils with rice and celery
green salad

Day Five
BREAKFAST
half a grapefruit
Muesli with low-fat milk
herbal tea
LUNCH
cream cheese and tomato sandwich with whole-grain bread
orange, peach, or nectarine
DINNER
mussels with white wine, garlic, and herbs
French bread
green salad

Day Six
BREAKFAST
melon and papaya fruit salad
2 slices of whole-grain toast with orange marmalade
herbal tea
LUNCH
mixed bean salad
French bread
DINNER
lamb chops
roasted eggplant and red pepper
tomato and onion salad

Day Seven

BREAKFAST

yogurt with mixed berries
2 slices of whole-grain toast
with honey

LUNCH

root vegetable soup
2 slices of rye bread

DINNER

grilled tuna with mashed potato
arugula, tomato, and cucumber salad
yogurt with honey and hazelnuts

HEALTHY SNACKS

Antioxidant-rich snacks can help to boost your intake. Keep some of the following handy for mid-morning or afternoon snacks.

piece of fresh fruit	fresh vegetables
small bowl of fruit salad	boiled egg
handful of dried fruit	small container of yogurt
handful of nuts	serving of frozen yogurt or ice cream
handful of seeds	piece of cheese
whole-grain bread	cup of tea
Melba toast	glass of freshly squeezed fruit juice
small bowl of cereal	glass of milk

Eating right
Antioxidants are present in many popular foods, including fruits, vegetables, poultry, meat, fish, and tea. They are easy to incorporate into a tasty, nutritious, and diverse diet—as here in grilled tuna with pesto mashed potato.

Taking care of your voice

Stressing your voice on a regular basis can damage the vocal cords, leading to permanent hoarseness. Furthermore, when the rest of your body is stressed, your voice can suffer. Learning to relax your voice is the key to keeping it healthy.

Stress can be thought of in two ways. Firstly, the emotional response to a situation can manifest itself in stress if there is a feeling of lack of control. This is the "fight-or-flight" response, which prepares your body for action. Whichever you choose, your voice may come into play. Shouting may increase the aggression, which is helping you fight, or tell that you are going to flee. Second, you can consciously choose to place your body under stress in order to maximize its response, for example when running a race or when singing an opera.

These are both examples of physiological stress, a condition that occurs when the body is asked to perform activities far outside of its regular functioning capacity. This is a situation that is often demanded of the voice—just think of the number of times in the past week that you have raised your voice louder than necessary in speech or in song—and it is harmful to the vocal cords.

INSTANT DAMAGE

Your vocal cords are highly sensitive in order to produce the range of sounds they do, and extreme stress can have an instant, and sometimes prolonged, effect on them.

Shouting down the house

When you shout with too much force, it is possible to damage the lining of your vocal cords, causing hoarseness. The muscles in your throat tighten, and breathing becomes shallower in reaction to the excessive tension. This results in more effort being exerted to recover your voice, which can make it worse. If the voice isn't given time to recover from stress—if you shout while your voice is still hoarse and your throat is still sore—you risk damaging the vocal cords still further. If you find yourself regularly shouting in anger or frustration, getting help to figure out what is stressing you makes more sense than risking your voice. People who regularly stress their voices may need speech therapy to train them away from poor voice habits.

Clearing your throat

A lot of people cough and clear their throats when they are stressed. If this is done too aggressively, it can also result in vocal cord damage. It is much better to try to relax your throat by swallowing and having sips of water instead.

Reflux

Stress can also result in acid reflux, in which stomach acid flows up toward the larynx, causing discomfort and sometimes a voice disorder. To reduce reflux, give your body enough time to digest food properly before rushing around, try not to eat hurriedly, and don't eat immediately before going to bed.

Sounding stressed

A stressed voice may sound more aggressive, inviting negative reactions from others, and breathing may become shallower as the pace of speaking gets quicker. If you can take the tension out of your voice, you're more likely to breathe better, produce more efficient speech, and get a better response.

LONG-TERM DAMAGE

Sometimes damage is the result of continuing an action without observing signals telling you to relax. These include hoarseness and sore throats, as well as tension in your body.

Roaring crowds
Persistent shouting can lead to the development of vocal cord nodules and a permanently hoarse or breathy voice.

EXERCISES TO RELAX A TENSE VOICE

1 Before working directly on your voice, focus on your whole body. Look for tension in your knees, back, abdomen, and face, all of which can accumulate to inhibit your natural ability to produce a healthy voice.

2 Now try an exercise from the Alexander technique. Lie on your back on the floor, support your head with a cushion or pillow, and bring your knees up, keeping your feet on the floor. Allow yourself to feel heavy, close your eyes, and focus on slow, gentle breathing. Try tensing and then letting go of different groups of muscles around your body to increase your awareness of tension. Now gently roll your head from side to side to release tension in your neck; this should make your voice feel freer and easier to use.

3 Sit upright in a chair and put one hand on your chest and one on your abdomen. Breathe in to the bottom of your lungs and feel both hands move out; if you find yourself gulping air, slow your breathing. Inhale through your nose as slowly as you can, aiming to get to the count of 10, then exhale just as slowly. If you hear a harsh whisper when you breathe in, you are narrowing your throat and tensing your vocal cords too much. This exercise should make you aware of the coordination between breathing and speaking.

4 Practise humming a single note. You should feel a buzzing sensation in your lips and eventually your face; if you can't feel it, try placing your fingers lightly over your face and nose. This encourages you to project your voice and to create greater resonance by taking the effort away from your vocal cords.

5 Try humming a continuous note while clenching your teeth. Your voice will sound trapped, thin, and nasal. Now start making a chewing motion, which relaxes the jaw, and notice how the sound becomes bigger and moves forward in your mouth.

Be career wise

Certain jobs carry greater risks for the voice than others. The traditional regimental sergeant major obviously stresses his voice on a daily basis, but singers, teachers, lawyers, clergymen, aerobics instructors, and politicians also regularly risk voice damage.

The problem is compounded in some cases by environmental factors: the atmosphere in many classrooms, for example, is dry, which is bad for the throat. In addition, many public buildings are built without the advice of an acoustician, so professionals may have to fill a space that was not designed for a single human voice. Noise, too, makes matters worse. Studies have shown that we tend to raise our voices by about 3 decibels for every 10 decibel increase in ambient noise level. Because the noise level in a kindergarten class can be as high as 80 decibels, it is not surprising that teachers suffer from voice problems.

If you belong to one of these at-risk groups, it's important to be especially kind to your larynx.

A survey found that although teachers make up only 4 percent of the U.S. work force, they make up 20 percent of patients at voice clinics.

Careful karaoke

Singers are prone to voice problems because of the extra effort they use in the throat when singing.

Professional singers are taught to warm their voices before rehearsing or performing, singing mid-range notes before gradually working toward those at the top and bottom of their ranges, and practicing scales and arpeggios, as well as breathing exercises to help in efficient, unstrained sound production.

Amateurs, however, may not take such care. Vocal difficulties often arise from a poorly produced loud voice, intended to fill a bar or concert hall. Such sounds can easily result in bruised vocal cords. It is wise not to sing without warming the voice as described above, especially if you have a sore throat, because you will be vulnerable to inflammation of the vocal cords.

Even with training, professionals face problems.

- Overuse of the vocal cords through extensive rehearsal and performance schedules.
- Travel, particularly by air, which is noisy and tiring, as well as involving sitting in a pressurized, low-humidity environment, can stress even a professional's voice.
- As with people who participate in sports, singers need to acclimatize to high altitudes before they can perform without risking voice stress.
- The atmosphere in many auditoriums is cold, dry, and dusty, which can harm the vocal cords.
- Some clubs and small venues allow smoking, which compromises performers' voices.

To club or not to club

If you are going out to a club or concert where the music is loud, accept that you are not going to be able to chat, too. Average noise levels are too loud to shout over. The

positive health tips

Be kind to your larynx: How to look after your voice

- If your job involves talking a lot, make sure you have quiet periods in the day.

- Don't talk above loud background noise if you don't have to.

- If you find you are often shouting as a way of dealing with anger, consider counseling or assertiveness training.

- Don't overdo spicy foods; they can cause laryngeal irritation.

- Steer clear of chemicals that might irritate your throat, such as aerosol sprays and household cleaning products.

- Avoid smoking and excessive drinking.

- Don't sit hunched over your computer keyboard or desk. This puts a strain on your neck muscles, which are important in voice production.

- Don't spend too long in cold, dry air. The larynx likes to be wet and warm. Steam inhalation will thin out mucus trapped in the nose and throat.

Controlling presence
Teachers who manage to maintain a disciplined atmosphere through their presence, rather than relying on shouting above the din of the playground, risk less voice stress than their colleagues.

atmosphere in such venues may be smoky, too, which will also affect your throat and voice.

Unclench that jaw
If you are overly tense, you may grind your teeth at night, resulting in a clenched jaw. This is another very common cause of vocal tension, making the voice sound "held back" or muffled. If you find yourself swallowing your sounds and having to make an extra effort with your throat to compensate for not being heard, you may need to take steps to undo the tension. We all clench our

jaws and grit our teeth when we are feeling stressed—the expression "grit your teeth" comes from having to restrain tension and frustration—but it should not become almost permanent.

Be socially wise
Two of the most common social stress relievers, smoking and alcohol, both dry out the voice and irritate the larynx, resulting in deepening, hoarseness, and other changes. Some people find this sexy—and some performers cultivate this style—but in the long run it ages the voice.

Keep lubricated
Stress can result in neglecting to eat when you need to or not drinking enough fluids throughout the day, which results in dehydration and a dry throat.

IT'S NOT TRUE!

"If the vocal cords are healthy, the voice is too."

Your voice does not depend solely on healthy vocal cords, but on a combination of three things working together. They are
• breathing, which provides the necessary power;
• the moving vocal cords, which are the source of the sound;
• your mouth and facial structures, which act as a filter, changing the size and shape of the sound.

If you spread your lips, your voice sounds brighter, whereas if you round them, it comes out deeper and duller.

Harmful habits

*Some of the lifestyle habits that many people consider
to be an integral part of a "normal" social life can seriously
damage your entire body, including your ears, nose,
and throat.*

Social drugs fall into two broad
categories: legal drugs such as
tobacco and alcohol, and illegal or
street drugs, including marijuana,
cocaine, and inhalants.

TOBACCO SMOKING
Smoking tobacco causes a
variety of disorders in the ears,
nose, and throat. These range
from relatively minor problems,
such as heavy snoring, to fatal
cancers of the nose and throat.
Choosing not to smoke can prevent
or significantly reduce the risk of
developing some of the following
health problems.

Airway damage
The airways from the nose and
mouth to the lungs are lined with a
layer of mucus that helps to keep
them clean and lubricated. This
mucus contains antibodies to kill
germs and is kept moving by a layer
of tiny hairlike tissues called cilia.
These hairs need a continuous supply
of oxygen to function properly, but
tobacco smoke restricts oxygen
supply, paralyzing the cilia so that
they no longer perform the essential
clearing action. Long-term smoking
makes the paralysis permanent, so
that mucus has to be coughed up. The
result is the typical "smoker's cough."

Coughs and colds
People who smoke are more
susceptible to coughs and colds
because the immune system is
harmed by tobacco smoke. For the

same reason, they often suffer worse
symptoms and take longer to get
over colds than nonsmokers.

Smoking is associated with an
increased risk of acute and chronic
rhinitis (inflammation of the mucus
membrane lining the nose). Smokers
are also at greater risk of sinusitis—
inflammation of the tissues lining the
sinus cavities—the condition often
improves if people stop smoking.

Snoring
Heavy smokers are more likely to
snore. Children exposed to
environmental tobacco smoke
(passive smoking) are also more
likely to snore, and the more smoke
they are exposed to, the greater the
likelihood they will snore. Experts
have found that if one parent
smokes, a child is roughly twice as

Understanding the risks
*Schools and youth and community groups
regularly invite police officers or counselors
from charitable organizations to discuss the
legal, social, and health implications of
drinking and drug use.*

likely to snore than if the parent
doesn't smoke, and if both parents
smoke, the child's risk of snoring
nearly quadruples.

Mouth and throat cancer
There is a strong association between
cancers of the mouth and throat and
smoking. It is estimated that about
85 percent of mouth and throat
cancers are caused by tobacco use,
and heavy use of both tobacco and
alcohol increases risk dramatically.
Tobacco smoke contains thousands
of different chemicals that are

Snoring affects 50 percent of men and 25 percent of women, most of them over age 40. Alcohol and obesity exacerbate the problem.

released into the air as particles and gases. At least 40 of these, including benzene, formaldehyde, and carbon monoxide, are known to cause cancer. Although some chemicals are present only in tiny quantities, the cumulative effect of inhaling this cocktail of toxic compounds causes cancer.

Although the lungs are the principal organs for the absorption of oxygen and other chemicals, some absorption also takes place in the nose and mouth. In fact, the nose is so efficient at absorbing substances into the bloodstream that some forms of medication are given in an aerosol formulation taken by nose.

Hearing loss
Smokers experience sudden hearing loss an average of 16 years earlier than people who have never smoked.

IT'S NOT TRUE!

"Smoking is safe if you don't inhale."

Cigarette smokers who do not inhale, as well as cigar and pipe smokers, often believe that their risk of cancer is minimized. It is true that these groups have a lower risk of lung cancer than cigarette smokers, but they are still twice as likely as nonsmokers to develop lung cancer. They also run a greater risk of mouth and throat cancer than lifelong nonsmokers.

In addition, smokers are more likely than nonsmokers to experience recurrent sudden hearing loss: 46 percent of smokers suffer such a recurrence, whereas just 33 percent of nonsmokers do.

Although experts are not sure how smoking increases a person's risk of hearing loss caused by exposure to loud noise, they believe decreased blood flow to the ears may play a role. The inner ear contains sensory cells and other tissues critical for hearing and the vessels that carry blood to the inner ear can become blocked by atherosclerosis (fatty plaques that adhere to the blood vessel walls). Furthermore, some researchers believe that high levels of carbon monoxide in the blood of smokers may directly damage sensory cells in the inner ear. Hearing loss is also directly related to aging, and although this type of loss is common, there is some evidence that smoking may accelerate it.

ALCOHOL AND THE BODY
Alcohol affects all the body systems, especially the brain and liver. Over-indulgence causes significant health hazards, but there could be some significant health benefits associated with low or moderate consumption.

Ear, nose, and throat damage
Alcohol consumption is associated with a number of cancers of the nose and throat, particularly in smokers. Alcohol is not a carcinogen in standard laboratory tests, but it may act as a "co-carcinogen" or tumor

---

Drinking to your health

Moderate alcohol consumption on a regular basis is considered by many to be beneficial to overall health. Experts argue about the definition of moderate consumption, but generally agree that one or two drinks per day, depending on your gender and body weight, seem to lessen the chances of coronary heart disease and cardiovascular disease. Evidence also seems to show that moderate drinking can reduce the risk of kidney stones and osteoporosis and help in the prevention of Alzheimer's disease.

... or ill health?

Studies suggest that drinking alcohol increases the risk of cancers of the mouth, pharynx, and larynx; the more consumed, the greater the risk. These risks are further multiplied by smoking: Drinking four units of alcohol a day doubles the risk of oral and pharyngeal cancer, but combined with 20 cigarettes a day, the risk is quadrupled. A person who smokes 40 cigarettes a day has 15 times the cancer risk of a nonsmoker and nondrinker.

promoter by irritating the lining of the gastrointestinal tract, making it more susceptible to the carcinogens in cigarette smoke.

ILLEGAL DRUGS

Illegal drug habits that are potentially damaging to the ears, nose, or throat include smoking marijuana, snorting cocaine, and inhaling solvents. Some of these drugs are harmful in the long term; others can do instant damage.

Marijuana

The harmful effects of smoking marijuana are similar to those of smoking tobacco, although people tend to smoke less marijuana than tobacco. Instant bodily reactions can be dry mouth, throat, nose, and eyes. Cancer is one possible form of permanent damage. Marijuana contains more carcinogens than

tobacco smoke, and more tar. It is also usually inhaled deeper into the lungs and held there longer. For these reasons, some experts consider it even more likely to cause cancer than tobacco smoke.

Cocaine

Cocaine can cause both temporary and permanent damage to the body, depending on the method of use.

Snorting cocaine is particularly harmful to the nose and throat. The drug is absorbed into the bloodstream through the nasal tissues, causing a stuffy or runny nose, sinus problems, loss of smell, chapped nostrils, nosebleeds, sores around the nostrils, difficulty swallowing, and hoarseness.

Prolonged snorting of cocaine can ulcerate the mucous membrane of the nose and damage the nasal septum, causing it to collapse. Because cocaine has anesthetic qualities, users may not even realize the damage being done to their noses and mouths.

Nose and throat symptoms of smoking cocaine include dry lips and throat, hoarseness, and a cough, which signals the damage being inflicted on the lungs.

Inhalants

An inhaled substance reaches the brain faster than anything that is injected, and the body's reaction to

Inadvertent damage
Many household products contain substances that produce a "high." If at all possible, use these products outdoors and wear a facemask to protect your nose and throat. If you must work indoors, ensure good ventilation.

Passive smoking

Children who are exposed to tobacco smoke are particularly susceptible to ear infections, which may in turn lead to deafness. They also have more sore throats, stuffy noses, hoarseness, and trouble getting over colds than other children, and they are more likely to require surgery to remove their adenoids and tonsils. Children of smokers are 30 to 80 percent more likely than children of nonsmokers to have chronic coughs or phlegm production. This is especially true for preschool children, who may spend more hours each day in a smoky environment.

inhalant fumes is potentially deadly. The immediate effects of inhalants on the nose and throat are caused by the body trying desperately to filter out the chemicals before they reach the lungs and brain. Such effects can include sneezing, coughing, nosebleeds, decreased sense of smell, and depressed breathing. Signs of solvent abuse include a red or running nose, sores around the mouth and nose, and bad breath.

Hundreds of substances can be inhaled. They include adhesives, aerosols such as spray paint and hair spray, and anesthetics such as nitrous oxide, or laughing gas, found in whipped cream cannisters. Cleaning products such as dry cleaning fluid or spot remover, and solvents such as nail polish remover, paint thinner and remover, and lighter fluid are also commonly abused substances.

Balancing acts

Good balance is essential in practically everything we do, from climbing stairs and lifting a child to riding a bike or carrying a cup of tea. Whatever your age, you can always improve your balance through regular exercise.

Like so many aspects of our health, we tend to take our sense of balance for granted, only noticing it when we experience problems. Both the ears and eyes play important roles in maintaining balance, sending different but complementary messages for the brain to interpret.

The balancing elite
Snowboarders require particularly good balance and coordination, attributes that combine to provide vital spatial awareness.

BALANCE AND SPORTS

If you exercise regularly, you are working on your balance without realizing it. Walking, using a treadmill, and riding a road bike all require balance and coordination; more obviously, activities such as yoga, ice skating, and skiing require good balancing skills. Sports scientists believe that the abilities to move and balance, as well as reaction times, are inextricably linked, and that all are crucial to successful sports performance.

If balance starts to become a problem, you should talk either to a fitness trainer at the local gym or to a physical therapist. Both of these professionals can devise a series of exercises or suggest sports activities to suit your balance problem, age, and state of health. There is no need to give up exercise.

WHEN BALANCE IS A PROBLEM

Everyday causes of dizziness, such as rapid head movement, motion sickness, and excess alcohol consumption, do not persist for long and are not necessarily causes for concern. There are more permanent causes of dizziness, however, that have lasting implications for well-being, and these include labyrinthitis, Meniere's disease, vertigo, and chronic middle ear infection. All of these require professional medical advice, and you should consult a doctor if you have prolonged dizziness with no obvious cause or if dizziness interferes with your regular daily routine.

If you have vertigo

For sufferers of vertigo and other vestibular complaints, there is a series of exercises that specifically address the problem of balance. The Cawthorne–Cooksey exercises, derived from British surgeon Terence

Cawthorne's research into balance and movement therapy in the 1940s, form the basis of accepted treatment for sufferers of dizziness. These exercises need to be repeated twice daily on a regular basis, and initially should be carried out under the supervision of a physical therapist.

positive health tips

Beating balance problems

- If you feel dizzy, hold on to something firm. Keep your eyes closed or focused on an immobile object and avoid moving your head.

- Your doctor may prescribe pills or shots to reduce signals traveling from the ears to the brain during a dizzy spell.

- Cut down on alcohol, caffeine, and salt. Although this does not help all forms of dizziness, it does reduce the severity of symptoms in many cases.

- Avoid stress. Find ways to deal with stressful situations, such as stress management techniques, or try yoga or meditation.

- Don't make radical lifestyle changes. Dizzy spells may mean that you need to curtail certain activities, but don't stop doing things you enjoy.

- Get support. There are many support groups, both local and on the Internet, for sufferers from chronic dizziness. Group members know how you feel and will have positive advice and tips to help you cope.

1

2

3

4

5a

5c

5b

Balance for all

These Cawthorne–Cooksey exercises, in addition to helping those with balance problems, are useful for anyone who wants to improve balance in general.

1 Walk up and down stairs carefully, with your eyes open and then repeat with your eyes closed. Hold on to a railing for safety, if needed, especially if your eyes are closed.

2 While standing, practice making sudden 90-degree turns, first with your eyes open and then with them closed.

3 Look side to side while walking. A supermarket is a good place to do this —read labels as you walk down the aisle.

4 Practice standing on one foot. Do this with your eyes open and then with them closed. Repeat with the other foot.

5 Stand on a soft surface such as a mattress, pillow, or foam mat.

a. First walk across the surface to get used to it.

b. Walk heel to toe across the surface, first with your eyes open and then with them closed.

c. Practice standing on one foot with your eyes open and then with them closed.

Stay healthy when exercising

All sports and activities, in moderation, are beneficial to your health and well-being, but there are some instances in which there are extra benefits for the ears, nose, and throat—and others in which it is advisable to take special care.

Many sports and exercise activities improve or help you maintain your balancing skills, but few specifically promote the health of your ears, nose, and throat. Exercise nonetheless is a great booster for the immune system, and will help to prevent the common, persistent, and sometimes painful infections that affect the ears, nose, and throat.

There are also some precautions and protective measures you should take when participating in some sports.

COLD WEATHER PRECAUTIONS

Starting to exercise outdoors in cold weather can cause problems for your ears, nose, and throat. An increased demand for oxygen can make you breathe more cold air in through your nose and mouth, triggering irritation. If the cold air hurts your throat, wrap a scarf over your nose and mouth until you are thoroughly warm. Protect your ears with a hat. If exercise-induced asthma is a problem, take every precaution and use your medication as indicated by your doctor.

WARM WEATHER PRECAUTIONS

Hot dry air not only dehydrates the body, it also dries out the mucous membrane of the nose, which may compromise the nose's ability to filter dust. Your throat too is likely to suffer in extremely dry weather. Drink water throughout any exercise session in hot dry weather.

WATER SPORTS

Frequent swimming and water sports can be problematic for the ears, particularly for children. The most common risk is swimmer's ear, an infection of the outer ear canal. Water enters the ear during swimming, carrying with it potentially damaging bacteria or fungus particles. The water usually drains and the ear dries, leaving no risk from microorganisms. When the water does not drain, however, the ear does not dry out properly, providing a perfect wet and warm breeding ground for bacteria.

The first indications of swimmer's ear are a general stuffy feeling accompanied by itching. As the symptoms continue to develop, the ear canal becomes swollen, and a thin milky discharge may appear. With full-blown swimmer's ear, the sufferer will feel pain, and the ear will be sensitive to the touch, particularly the cartilage in front of the ear canal.

A chill in the air
Modern thermal headwear uses lightweight materials that breathe, allowing you to cover your nose and throat when you need to.

Are nose dilator strips effective?

TALKING POINT

Nose dilator strips have become almost ubiquitous in the sports world, especially among football players. The theory is that they make breathing easier by widening the nostrils, but their effectiveness has not been scientifically proven. In fact, it seems more likely that proper breathing techniques are responsible for improved performance, but the psychological effect of wearing these strips should not be underestimated. They have become so common that athletes who do not wear them may feel like they are at a disadvantage to those who do.

If you develop swimmer's ear, you should stop swimming and consult a doctor. You may be prescribed antibiotics or eardrops to clear up the infection, or it may resolve itself with time. Be careful not to get any water in your ears when bathing or showering for as long as the infection lasts.

When you do resume swimming, be cautious of how much water gets into the ear. Wearing earplugs can help, so ask your pharmacist or lifeguard for advice on the most suitable type for you. Finally, dry your ears thoroughly after swimming. To do this, either shake your head gently from side to side, or use alcohol eardrops (available from pharmacies). These evaporate excess water.

Pools and your health

It is important to remember that although chlorine kills many bacteria and viruses, it does not sterilize a swimming pool. In very hot weather, chlorine is less stable, and greater numbers of people are likely to be using the swimming pool. Infections of the nose and ears, as well as of the eyes—if you are not wearing goggles—can all be passed on.

EQUALIZING THE PRESSURE

Scuba diving (scuba stands for "self-contained underwater breathing apparatus") allows you to go far deeper under water than unassisted diving. The deeper you go, the greater the pressure of the water environment, the effects of which are felt mostly by the ears. As your body tries to adjust to the changing pressure, you will feel an increasing need to make your ears pop, or to "equalize" (see page 62). The

Self-protection
Many rugby players protect their heads with strong helmets; this should reduce the incidence of cauliflower ear among players, and it helps avert potential brain damage.

inability to do so should be taken very seriously, because the result could be a ruptured eardrum. This is particularly likely in divers suffering from colds or allergies.

CONTACT SPORTS

Activities such as boxing and rugby and other contact sports can be hazardous for the ears and nose. Although the practice turning and moving undoubtedly helps balance and coordination, boxers and rugby players suffer more broken noses and deformed, or cauliflower, ears than any other groups of athletes. If you intend to box or play rugby or any other contact sport, use every safety protection available and get any injury attended to as a medical emergency.

If you have suffered any injury to your nose and ears, avoid all contact sports until given the go-ahead by your doctor.

ENVIRONMENTAL RISK FACTORS

Every day, in our homes, workplaces, and the outside atmosphere, substances that are potentially harmful to the ears, nose, and throat abound. Knowing the risks and taking sensible precautions can go a long way to keeping these parts of the body healthy and functioning well.

80 *Noise is not only one of life's biggest stressors —it can also seriously damage hearing. Learn how to minimize the risks.*

85 *Being aware of the pollutants in every breath that meets your nose and throat is an important step to health.*

87 *Even our homes can compromise our health. Discover ways to avoid the majority of household ENT irritants.*

91 *Even if you suffer from allergies, gardening need not be off limits—if you take some simple precautions and choose your time wisely.*

Noise pollution

Because the damage that is done to hearing is invisible and is often only detected years later, we tend not to notice that it is being harmed. It is a fact, however, that hearing is easy to damage instantly and in the long term.

The human auditory system has evolved over millions of years to allow humans to extract the maximum amount of useful information from the environment, and this is all entirely beneficial. As in many other fields, however, industrial progress has brought with it a number of problems, including:

- The risk of occupational hearing loss for people working in industrial situations that are so noisy that normal speech and other natural sounds are drowned out.
- An ability to create louder and louder sounds through advances in amplification technology.

- The risk of severe annoyance, sleep disturbance, and psychological stress for people living close to main roads, airports, railways, and industrial and commercial sites, as well as those who have inconsiderate neighbors.

We all need to be aware of these risks, but we should not blow them out of proportion.

GOOD SOUND, BAD SOUND

For most people most of the time, the sounds around them are cause for celebration—life would be infinitely less rewarding if we couldn't hear speech, music, and the sounds of nature. However, sound does have properties that, in excess, can damage human hearing.

Sound waves

Sound consists of vibrating waves that reach the ears. These waves have two essential characteristics: amplitude, which is the loudness or volume of a sound, and frequency, which is its pitch.

> *Only 15 minutes of exposure a day to the noise level of a rock concert can damage hearing.*

In order for your ear to detect sound waves, the volume must be high enough to move the eardrum— inside of which are the tiny bones that convert the sound waves into mechanical vibrations. The vibrations are then converted to nerve impulses by the stereocilia and sent to the brain for interpretation (see page 24).

From safe to harmful

The human ear can pick up an incredible range of volumes. The lowest sound level on the decibel (dB) scale, 0 dB, is the level of the quietest sound pressure that anybody with so-called normal hearing can hear. Continuous exposure to sounds of 85–90 dB and more can damage hearing.

60 to 65 dB—normal conversational speech about 1 yard away

80 dB—loud music from the radio

90 dB—motorcycle, rush-hour city traffic

95 dB—chainsaw in operation

100–110 dB—small firecrackers, thunderstorm

On the other hand, the noise must not be so loud that it perforates the eardrum or damages the stereocilia.

For your ears to pick up sound waves, not only do the waves have to be of a certain volume, but they must also be within a range of frequency that is capable of stimulating the stereocilia in the cochlea. The extent of the human hearing range is 20 to 20,000 Hertz (Hz), but different people are sensitive to different frequencies.

NOISE AND YOUR HEALTH

Sound can be dangerous to the human body in two ways. First, loud noise has the potential to cause physical damage to the ear, which can result in hearing problems. Second, prolonged noise can produce emotional distress. Most people would agree that noise pollution is at best extremely annoying and at worst painful to the ear. Although the evidence is inconclusive, it seems that it may also have an impact on your health.

Physical damage

Loud noise is one of your ears' greatest enemies. The ears are extremely sensitive, and damage to any part of their structure can cause problems. Such damage is caused by either prolonged exposure to a loud noise or by a sudden noise. Damage can be permanent or temporary, and repeated instances of temporary harm may cause permanent damage. Damage to the ears doesn't necessarily mean hearing loss: Ringing in the ears and physical or psychological sensitivity to some sounds are also classified as ear damage.

- **Tinnitus** Tinnitus is persistent ringing in the ears that can be caused by very loud noise such as that at a nightclub or rock concert. In these instances, tinnitus usually only lasts a few hours and normal hearing returns, but it can be an ongoing condition. It also causes hyperacusis, extreme sensitivity to sound, in about 40 percent of tinnitus sufferers. Tinnitus is

What is a decibel?

A decibel is a measure of the intensity of sound, expressed as power per unit of surface area. The hearing level (or HL) scale starts on the threshold of human hearing, 0 dB, and extends upward. The threshold of pain is about 130 dB. Like the Richter scale, which measures earthquakes, the decibel scale is logarithmic, with a base of 10. This means that 10 dB is ten times louder than 0 dB; 20 dB is ten times louder than 10 dB (10 x 10) and 30 dB is ten times louder than 20 dB (10 x 10 x 10).

common in people with hearing loss, but people with "normal" hearing can also suffer from it.

- **Temporary hearing loss** This is the feeling of slight deafness you feel when you leave a rock concert, for

120 dB—amplified rock band, pneumatic road drill

127 dB—class of 30 children shouting as loudly as they can

130 dB—ambulance siren

140 dB—gunshot at close range, sandblasting

150 dB—jet engine on take-off; the space shuttle launch is louder still

example. Your hearing will recover from this trauma, but when it does depends on how long you were listening and how loud the music was.

- **Permanent hearing loss** Permanent hearing loss may be gradual, caused by exposure to noise over a period of time. This is sometimes referred to as occupational hearing loss. Like age-related hearing loss, it initially occurs in only a narrow band of frequencies, which widens with repeated exposure. Acoustic trauma is the instant loss of hearing caused by a short, very loud noise. This type of hearing loss is often more pronounced in the ear closest to the noise, which can affect your ability to perceive sounds or your ability to analyze sounds reaching the ears.

HOW NOISY IS TOO NOISY?

The National Institute for Deafness and Other Communication Disorders (NIDCD) gives the following guidelines for protecting your hearing.

- No more than 15 minutes of unprotected exposure to sounds above 100 decibels is recommended.
- Regular exposure lasting longer than 1 minute to sounds over 110 decibels can cause permanent hearing loss.
- Even one-time exposure can cause permanent hearing loss.

The NIDCD advises that sounds over 85–90 decibels have the potential to damage your ears. This is about the same decibel level as a lawn mower.

Number 1—42 percent of complaints are about amplified music: Practice unplugged if you can.

DIY causes 2 percent of complaints: Work during the day, if possible.

TV and radio make up 2 percent of complaints: Keep the volume down at night.

Domestic appliances cause noise and vibration and are run at inappropriate times.

PSYCHOLOGICAL STRESS

Several factors, including sleep disturbance, anger, and modified social behavior, have been attributed to noise pollution.

Stressed out

Your body responds automatically to noise in various ways. Most of these responses are completely normal and not necessarily harmful. People who are continually exposed to potentially threatening noises adapt to them, but may start to anticipate them. In theory at least, in susceptible individuals, this can lead to a chronic buildup of stress hormones and psychological anxiety. This has an impact on quality of life and may adversely affect an individual's long-term health.

Noisy nights

Evidence suggests that most people adapt to noise at night or at least change their behavior to compensate in some way. Electroencephalogram (EEG) measurements show harmless neural responses to familiar noises while subjects sleep, only a small proportion of which go on to cause any measurable disruption to the normal pattern of sleep. This might be a change from a deeper to a lighter stage of sleep, sometimes even leading to awakening, but contrary to the general impression given by complaints about sleep disturbances caused by noise, it is remarkable how few noise events actually cause any measurable or significant disruption. Problems occur when

After general domestic noise (number two), barking dogs come in at number three: Don't leave a dog alone in a house or garden.

Noisy neighbors
Some local authorities publish lists of "noisy neighbor" complaints. Almost all sources of irritating noise can be avoided.

the noise is particularly loud or unexpected (such as a sudden thunderstorm), intermittent, or unfamiliar to your brain.

In addition, there may be individuals who cannot help anticipating the noise, thereby magnifying their anxiety and response. This can cause wakefulness and even sleep deprivation, which has an adverse effect on health.

WHAT YOU CAN DO

Minimizing noise pollution can be difficult, particularly in the case of acoustic trauma, because loud noises are often impossible to predict, so you cannot take steps to protect yourself. Despite this, the key to looking after your ears and reducing noise-related stress is to understand when you are in damaging environments and either alleviate the source or take protective measures.

At home

Although our homes are quieter than the outside world, there are still steps you can take to protect your ears.

- **TV, radio, and sound systems** Keep noise at a reasonable level: You should be able to talk easily over any piece of equipment. Be careful of the volume coming out of headphones and of that in confined spaces like your car. This also helps neighborly relations.
- **Home improvement** If you are using noisy equipment, make sure you protect your ears. This also applies to using garden equipment.

- **Sports and leisure** Your hobbies may be putting your ears at risk. Anyone who rides a motorbike or goes skeet shooting should wear ear protection.

At work

Not all jobs are located in obviously noisy environments, but it pays to be vigilant. Noise levels in restaurant kitchens, for example, can be high at busy times, and telemarketers may be exposed to loud noise through their headsets if these have not been fitted with volume-limiting devices.

- **Machinery** Workplaces with operating machinery are usually among the loudest. Garages, factories, construction sites, and road construction are obvious examples. Agricultural workers and horticulturists may also be at risk.
- **Music** Consider noise levels if you work in an environment where

FOR THE UNDER-12-YEAR-OLDS

Children and noise

Two recent studies have looked at the effect of airport noise on children. In Munich, Germany, more than 200 children were tested for blood pressure and levels of stress hormones six months before and six months after the opening of a new international airport. The second study looked at children living near the JFK International Airport in New York.

Although the results were not wholly conclusive in either test, children who lived under the flight path in Munich were shown to have higher blood pressure and levels of stress hormones than those who did not. (The two groups of children matched in terms of other factors, such as age, parental occupation, and socioeconomic status.)

Higher blood pressure and levels of stress hormones may be related to heart problems and elevated cholesterol levels in adulthood. The New York study found some evidence that children near the airport did not read or listen as well as children from other areas of the city.

Musical chairs

Musicians may suffer trauma to their ears if seated too close to the noisiest instruments, often the brass and percussion sections. Although earplugs may be available, some musicians find that playing while wearing them is not easy.

music is always playing, such as record stores, some bars, and sports arenas.

• Transportation Jet engines are among the biggest noisemakers, so airport workers must be especially vigilant. All city traffic contributes to noise levels, so anyone who works in city streets should take care. Employers are legally required to protect you when you are at work, and this includes your hearing. Your employer should have practices in place to assess the level of noise in all areas. If this level exceeds 85 decibels, you should be aware of the risks to your hearing, noisy areas should be clearly marked with warning signs, and you should be provided with protection for your ears. If you work

in a noisy environment, employers are required to have your hearing tested and monitored by experts.

Employees have responsibilities as well. Everyone should evaluate his or her individual exposure to noise, and if necessary take precautions. Failing to protect your ears if you work for extended periods in a noisy environment will cause cumulative and thus permanent damage. This will also happen if your ear protection doesn't fit properly. Check this by listening to your voice, which should sound louder and deeper if your protection is working properly. Short breaks are also beneficial.

Out and about

It is almost impossible to predict noises in the environment, but being aware of the risk may help you to minimize exposure. Be sure to wear earplugs at rock concerts and in nightclubs. If a movie theater's sound system hurts your ears, ask if it can be turned down. If not, leave.

What ear protection is available?

Two types of headgear protect the eardrums—earmuffs and earplugs. Both decrease the volume of sound allowed to reach your middle ear by sealing off the ear canal. Whether you choose earmuffs or earplugs, they will only be of use if they fit properly and thus reduce noise by 15 to 30 dB. Good-quality earplugs and earmuffs offer approximately equal sound reduction, although earplugs are considered better for low-frequency noise and earmuffs for high-frequency noise. Using both types of protection at once will reduce noise by a further 10 to 15 dB and should be considered in high-risk areas.

ASK THE EXPERT

Knowing the atmospheric irritants

Atmospheric pollution is all around us—in our homes, in workplaces, and outdoors. Increasing concentrations may mean that your nose and throat need a helping hand defending themselves.

The environment is full of chemicals and gases, as well as naturally occurring irritants. Symptoms that are slow to clear, such as a stuffy head, itchy throat, or runny nose, may be an indication of atmospheric irritants in your environment.

TYPES OF POLLUTION

There are two main types of airborne irritants that can adversely affect your health:

- Toxic air pollutants, including gases and vapors such as carbon monoxide, as well as petrochemical fumes, for example from household cleaning products
- Particulate matter, including dust and dust mites, and pollen from trees, shrubs, and flowers

These airborne pollutants can cause a number of temporary ailments when inhaled. Most—including a runny nose and itchy throat—occur in the nose and throat. In many cases, these symptoms are temporary, but they may signal potential long-term damage being done to the body. Just as even the best strainer on the market allows some impurities into your cooking, so the nose cannot filter out 100 percent of pollutants, particularly when the particles or atoms are too small to be trapped. Toxic airborne pollutants can be poisonous in small or large doses, instantly and over time.

TOXIC AIR POLLUTANTS

There are many sources of toxic pollutants in the environment. A number of them irritate the nose and throat, and all increase your risk of lung or bronchial disease, paralysis, or seizures. These fall into two groups: gases, vapors and fumes; and petrochemicals. These groupings make them easier to identify in, and eventually eradicate from, your environment (see pages 88–89 for tips on a healthy home).

- **Gases, vapors, and fumes** Gases such as carbon monoxide are exceedingly dangerous at high levels. Other harmful gases include carbon dioxide and sulfur dioxide. These may irritate your nose and throat, but their main damage is to the lungs, where they can severely impede breathing and cause respiratory paralysis.

Fresh country air?
Most people assume that country air is less polluted than city air. This is largely true, but there are still risks that must be controlled, such as spraying of agricultural chemicals.

Pets and allergies
Recent studies suggest that pets may not always be off limits for children with allergies. One study that followed children from birth to the age of seven found that those born into a household where there was already a cat or dog were less likely to suffer allergies than other children.

• Petrochemicals Petrochemicals are organic compounds found in many manufactured products. They can become dangerous if fumes accumulate and can affect the mucous membranes in the eyes, mouth, throat, and lungs. They also increase the risk of cancer.

PARTICULATE MATTER

Particulate matter irritates the nose and throat. This is not only because these body parts are in charge of filtering out airborne particles; it is also due to the allergic reactions such particles can trigger.

Eighty-five percent of children with allergic asthma are sensitive to dust mites.

Symptoms of an allergic reaction include sneezing, a runny or stuffy nose, watery and itchy eyes, and, possibly, headaches. Some allergies can also trigger asthma. Those who suffer from allergies are often sensitive to a number of allergens, and some of the most common are dust, pet hair and dander, and mold.

The demon dust and dust mites

Dust is not just dirt and grime; it includes a mixture of particles of skin, pet hair, food, clothing, and furnishings. Dust also contains microscopic dust mites that thrive in the warm, humid conditions found in modern buildings. It is mainly the fecal matter of these dust mites that triggers the allergic reactions that cause respiratory problems, including asthma and inflammation of the mucous membranes. Dust mites live in upholstery, carpets, and bedding.

Pollen

The seasonal type of allergic rhinitis is called hay fever and is most commonly caused by a reaction to pollen released by grasses, flowers, and trees. Pollen is the microscopic grains that plants manufacture to reproduce. Certain types of pollen are small, dry, light grains that travel very effectively in the air. It is predominantly these types that are referred to as atmospheric irritants, and that play havoc with the sinuses of hay fever sufferers.

Mold is also something to watch out for in the garden. The mold itself and the spores it produces can both cause allergic rhinitis.

Treatments

The most common treatment for allergic rhinitis is the prescription of antihistamine tablets, as well as the use of steroid inhalers and nasal sprays to help reduce inflammation and swelling. Alternative therapies are also popular with allergy sufferers (see pages 57–58). The most effective remedy, however, is to reduce the number of airborne irritants in your environment.

What is allergic rhinitis?

Allergic rhinitis occurs when your immune system overreacts to a foreign substance, such as pollen or dust, that does not bother most people. In such cases, the body manufactures elevated levels of an antibody called immunoglobulin E (IgE). Each IgE antibody binds to a specific allergen. When the two bind together, they stimulate the body's mast cells to release strong inflammatory chemicals, such as histamine.

ASK THE EXPERT

A healthy home and garden

Our homes and gardens are our last refuge from the stresses of the world, but they are not always safe havens. Both indoor and outdoor air can be polluted and may have a serious effect on your nose and throat.

INDOOR AIR QUALITY

Creating a home that is relatively free of airborne pollutants takes effort, but with time and care, you will soon notice an improvement in the symptoms of exposure to atmospheric irritants, such as a runny nose, sneezing, and sore throat.

GAS, VAPOR, AND FUME-FREE LIVING

It is important to eliminate or reduce fumes and toxic gases. To do this, check the services coming into the building, especially gas pipes, for leaks. If you have a choice, build a garage separate from the house, or keep the connecting door to the house closed so that exhaust fumes do not get into the house. Check that gas from ovens and heaters is properly vented to the outside—never use a gas heater in a closed room. When buying a new fireplace or restoring an old one, install a sealed primary or secondary combustion stove. These are energy efficient and environment-friendly.

Eliminating petrochemicals

Petrochemicals give off fumes and are found in an enormous number of products in our homes. Synthetic carpets and padding, in particular, are laden with them. To reduce petrochemical fumes, replace your carpet with floorboards or coverings made from natural fibers such as wool, jute, sea grass, or coconut. The furnishings and fabrics in your home may also have been chemically treated and can emit fumes. The best replacements for these materials are organic natural fibers that have not been bleached or treated, including linen or cotton.

Many chemical irritants are found in ordinary household cleaners, especially those for ovens, carpets, windows, and upholstery. Formaldehyde, phenols, ammonia, and chlorine are found in bleaches, disinfectants, detergents, air fresheners, and personal hygiene products and have all been found to increase health risks. Symptoms include inflammation of mucous membranes, nasal congestion, upper respiratory tract infection, nausea, headaches, and eye irritation.

What are the irritants?

When purchasing products, read the labels to see what you are getting. If you can't avoid irritant chemicals, be careful not to breathe in their fumes.

ACETONE (nail polish remover)
nose, throat, eye, and lung irritation; headaches, dizziness

AMMONIA (household cleaners)
breathing problems

BENZENE (dyes, detergents)
headaches, dizziness, nausea, and breathing problems

ETHYL ALCOHOL (antifreeze)
eye irritation, breathing problems, headaches, drowsiness

ETHYL ACETATE (printing inks)
anemia; eye, nose, and gum irritations; breathing problems, lethargy

FORMALDEHYDE (fiberboard)
breathing problems; eye, ear, and nose irritation

METHYL ALCOHOL (solvents)
headaches, nausea, irritation of mucous membranes

TOLUENE (paint, paint thinners)
impaired coordination, mental sluggishness, loss of hearing and vision

TRICHLOROETHYLENE (degreasers)
headaches, dizziness, memory loss, breathing problems

XYLENE (paint, paint thinners)
nausea, coughs, inflammation of mucous membranes, nose and throat irritation

KEEPING MITES AT BAY

Dust mites are inevitable in today's homes. They provoke irritation of the nasal passages and eyes and are the major cause of asthma symptoms in many sufferers. Controlling the number of them in your home needs a regular and methodical approach. Here are eight tips to get you started.

PROTECT YOUR BEDDING
Cover your mattress, quilt, and pillows with a dust mite–proof cover.

WASH BEDDING IN HOT WATER
Washing bed covers, sheets, and pillow cases at 140°F removes mites and their droppings.

VENTILATE
Thoroughly ventilating the house by opening the windows helps to prevent dampness.

VACUUM REGULARLY
Vacuuming daily with an efficient vacuum cleaner and damp dusting pick up mites and their droppings.

MAKE YOUR HOME A DUST-FREE ZONE

It is unrealistic to expect to get rid of all airborne irritants in our homes, but we can do a great deal to reduce dust. Living in a dust-free zone will have a dramatic effect on your health even if you do not suffer from allergies or asthma.

Remove clutter from windowsills and tabletops, especially knicknacks, picture frames, books, and magazines, which collect a great deal of dust. Open the windows and thoroughly air out your home, and then dust all surfaces well. It is a good idea to use an electrostatically charged cloth, which will pick up the dust without rereleasing it into the air.

Wash your curtains and loose soft furnishings using a detergent made from natural products. Vertical blinds will collect less dust than traditional curtains, swags and drapes, or venetian blinds.

Carpets hold and release dust. If you want to keep your carpeting, replace synthetic carpets and padding with those made from natural fibers. Vacuum them well and, if possible, get them steam-cleaned using eco-friendly products that do not contain chemical irritants. Ideally, you should replace carpets with a solid floor covering. The more flat, even, and smooth floor surfaces you have in your home, the less opportunity there is for dust to build up. For this

IT'S NOT TRUE!

"Short-haired breeds do not cause allergies."

The problem with hairy or furry pets is not their hair or fur. It is their dander, microscopic particles of dead skin, and saliva that provoke symptoms. Despite evidence to the contrary from asthma sufferers, research has shown that short-haired pets are as much of a problem as long-haired ones. Even hairless breeds can provoke asthma symptoms or allergic reactions.

FREEZE SOFT TOYS
Placing soft toys in the freezer for 24 hours every two weeks kills mites, which can then be removed by washing in hot water.

PREVENT STATIC
Dry your clothing and laundry outside whenever possible (unless you suffer from hay fever).

AIR OUT BEDDING
Air out your bedding regularly, especially in winter, when homes tend to be less well ventilated.

PREVENT DUST BUILDUP
Replace carpets with a smooth finish timber or other even floor surface, such as vinyl.

There are more than 2 million dust mites in the average double mattress.

reason, smooth timber floors are recommended for anyone who regularly suffers from asthma or other allergies.

Vacuum frequently, especially where there is carpet. If your vacuum cleaner has a filter, make sure you change it regularly, and if any member of the household is particularly sensitive to dust, you may consider buying a vacuum cleaner fitted with high-efficiency particulate air filters.

Do not allow pets into bedrooms; some of their allergens are carried on very small particles and will remain airborne for long periods.

Pet dander is difficult to remove from carpets and furnishings and easily transfers onto clothes. Restricting your pet's access to some areas of the house will dramatically reduce the level of allergen exposure. You can further minimize the problem by having your pet regularly washed and groomed. If anyone in your home keeps rabbits, rats, guinea pigs, or gerbils, keep them in a secure hutch away from the house.

Desensitization treatment may have benefits, so it is worth discussing this option with your specialist.

OTHER MEANS AND METHODS

In addition to reducing the pollutants and irritants that enter your home, there is plenty you can do to minimize the impact of substances that are already present and are difficult to eliminate.

Ventilation

It is only natural to want to be warm and dry in the home in winter, but lack of proper ventilation can cause health problems. Like you, your house needs to breathe, and it does this through the walls as well as through doors and windows. Dust and pollution soon build up inside a sealed house. Damp and humid

Water feature

If you do not want to buy an ionizer, there is a natural alternative. Moving water creates negative ions, so a small indoor water feature or pebble fountain will naturally ionize the air.

What does an ionizer do?

In a natural, clean, outdoor environment, the electrostatic balance of positive and negative ions in the air is approximately equal. Inside a building, however, the negative ions are depleted by many aspects of daily living, such as breathing, heating, air conditioning, and computers. This imbalance causes the positively charged ions to attract and hold dust particles and can cause various health problems, including allergies. An ionizer works to restore electrical balance.

ASK THE EXPERT

conditions encourage mold to form, and create an environment in which dust mites flourish. If your house feels damp, check for leaks and moisture. It may be that moisture is trapped inside a cavity wall, in which case you will need professional advice on what you can do to help it escape so that your house can dry out. Removing leaks and moisture from your home can be a tall order.

Most modern homes are finished with nonporous paints, which trap moisture inside. A dehumidifier can regulate excess moisture but does not necessarily solve the problem. One solution is to strip nonporous paint and repaint the inside and outside of your house with porous paint, which allows the water inside to evaporate into the air outside.

Air conditioning

Air conditioning systems contain filters that reduce the number of airborne pollutants brought into the home from outside. Air conditioning also reduces the humidity in the air

that circulates, which cuts down on potential molds and fungi. However, poor maintenance leads to a less efficient system and can provide a perfect breeding ground for airborne diseases, which may then be distributed throughout the air-conditioned environment.

Air filters

When choosing an air filter, you should make sure that it is a high-efficiency particulate air filter, and keep in mind that the greater the surface area of the filter, the more effectively it will work. Such filters have been shown to benefit people with asthma and allergy sufferers, and are often combined with an activated carbon filter to clear chemical pollution from the air.

Electrostatic filters

These are generally useful in filtering smoke and other larger particulate matter but are less effective for smaller particles such as airborne bacteria and viruses, gases, and odors. This restricts their usefulness to allergy sufferers.

Air ionizers

Simple ionizers draw in air and give dust particles a negative charge so that dirt is pulled out of the air and onto the nearest relatively positively charged surface, from which it can easily be cleaned. Electrostatic filters also ionize air passing through them but contain a positively charged filter to collect the dust particles as they pass through the device, resulting in cleaner air.

There is evidence, however, that ionizers can increase some symptoms, such as nighttime cough.

When springtime isn't fun

During the onset of spring and its progression to summer, there is a general pattern to the order in which species pollinate. This pattern can help sufferers to avoid certain triggers.

A HEALTHY GARDEN

Although you can't eliminate all the airborne pollutants from the outdoor environment, you can significantly reduce their concentration in your own garden.

GARDEN IRRITANTS

Two of the biggest garden irritants to your nose and throat are pollen from trees, flowers, grass, and weeds, and spores from molds and fungi growing in rotting vegetation.

Mold spores are the reproductive particles of mold. Each spore can give rise to a new mold that can produce millions more spores. Both the spores and tiny fragments of mold can cause allergic rhinitis if they are inhaled.

People who suffer from allergic rhinitis (hay fever) are sensitive to pollen and molds and can have acute symptoms including a runny or stuffy nose, inflammation of the nose and throat, irritation of the eyes, and inflammation of the sinuses.

IF YOU HAVE ALLERGIES

Carefully monitoring pollen levels, taking preventive and protective measures, and avoiding plants that release pollen into the air can minimize problems and let you enjoy your garden.

Pollen levels

Pollen levels are widely monitored and many local news agencies offer daily pollen count indexes,

APRIL/MAY
Most sufferers begin to experience symptoms at the start of spring, and it is the wind-pollinated trees that produce the greatest amounts of airborne pollen at this time. Among the first species to pollinate are alder and elm.

JUNE/JULY
The plant species to avoid at the height of spring and early summer are many and varied. They include spring-flowering weeds, rye grass, and most trees. Highly scented plants can also trigger hay fever and, depending on their species, may be blooming at this time.

AUGUST
August is generally considered the worst month for hay fever sufferers in the United States. This is mostly because pollen, which is responsible for 90 percent of all allergic rhinitis, is at its peak in August.

SEPTEMBER
In September, ragweed is the mostly likely cause of allergic rhinitis. Mold spores also are often airborne during summer months and into autumn, when things become damp.

particularly during the spring and summer months. The Weather Channel and AccuWeather websites also give national and local pollen forecasts. When levels are expected to be exceptionally high, remain indoors if possible. Keep an eye on local weather conditions, too, and use them to your benefit.

- Early morning rain prevents the release of pollen that day, so allergies should not be a problem on those days; rain later in the day washes pollen from the air.
- Wind stirs up pollen and dust, so take every precaution on blustery days; similarly, on hot, still days, pollen "hangs" in the air.
- Sunny days raise pollen to cloud level during the morning, and it

Does wearing a mask protect my nose from pollen?

Wearing a face mask on days when the pollen count is high can drastically reduce the irritating particles entering your nose, as long as you follow instructions on changing and cleaning the filter. The best types of mask are those made from an electrostatically charged material that filters out very small particles down to 0.04 of a micron. This gives much better protection than an ordinary face mask, which only filters out larger particles. A scarf or handkerchief will provide hardly any protection at all, because the pollen and dust particles are small enough to pass through the weave of the fabric.

ASK THE EXPERT

only falls when the temperature starts to drop. Do any gardening in the early morning or afternoon, or restrict it to cool, cloudy days.

Mowing the lawn

It is best to mow the lawn in the early morning, ideally while there is still a little dew to dampen things down. Regular trimming is a good idea, and it is better to use a rotary mower rather than an electric-powered one to restrict blowing the grass cuttings around (a machine with a bag to collect the clippings is best). Close the windows of the house before mowing and for some time after.

All gardeners with allergies must pay careful attention to their clothes. Wear a long-sleeved shirt, hat, gloves, and dark glasses to avoid eye and skin contact with plants that could cause an allergic reaction. A mask made specifically for this is useful. After being outdoors, shower to wash off the pollen that will have collected on your clothes and body and in your hair. Don't wear your gardening clothes in the house.

Weeding

Hoeing is more sensible than weeding, if you can keep weeds under control in this way, because your nose and eyes are further away from the plants. Planting good ground cover can reduce or even eliminate the need for weeding. Low-allergen ground cover plants that also suppress weeds include periwinkle, common bugle, bellflower (campanula), plantain lily, and ferns. Covering any unplanted areas with plastic sheeting or gravel mulch can also suppress weeds.

Choosing plants wisely

Plants vary in the amount of pollen they produce and the method they use to distribute it. Gardeners with hay fever should try to avoid wind-pollinated plants.

Wind-blown pollen is small, light, and easily spread. Even if you are not allergic to pollen you could become sensitized by breathing it in, especially in large quantities. Wind-pollinated plants include all grasses, many trees, and some wildflowers. Avoid such trees as ash, birch, elder, hazel, horse chestnut, oak, willow, and yew.

A high-pollen tree in your garden exposes you to 10 times more pollen than a similar tree a block away.

Choose insect-pollinated plants instead; these produce heavier, stickier pollen, which is less likely to be released into the air. Most shrubs and flowers with large petals are insect pollinated, as are most herbs. Blossom trees are also generally pollinated by insects.

Try to avoid heavily scented flowers, which may trigger asthma. These include freesia, jasmine, and wisteria. Even lightly scented plants can harbor wind-blown pollen, so it's best not to smell them.

The good news is that many of the brightest colored flowers are showy precisely to attract pollinating insects, so these can form a major feature of your garden. Plants to choose include clematis, irises, and violas, as well as such popular annuals as snapdragons, impatiens, and cornflowers.

Hedges can give rise to mold and spores. Replace them with fences or brick walls.

Don't plant vines too close to the house, where their scent can drift through open windows.

Make the most of moisture-loving pool and marginal plants, which do not usually cause allergies.

Select insect-pollinated rather than wind-pollinated species.

Dampen the air by adding a water feature to your garden, but avoid fountains that make pollen and spores airborne.

CREATING A LOW-ALLERGEN GARDEN

In addition to the points illustrated, take note of the following factors when creating a low-allergen garden.

- Avoid compost heaps and piles of logs, which can harbor mold spores.
- Try not to use heavily scented plants.
- Mulch with gravel or pebbles: Hay, straw, and bark chips may harbor molds and spores.
- Create a paved area close to the house and minimize the size of your lawn.

Use low-allergen ground cover plants such as periwinkle and hosta to suppress weeds.

3

What happens
when things go wrong

Knowing what can go wrong

Almost everyone has had an ailment affecting the ears, nose, or throat at some stage in his or her life. People of all ages are susceptible, and there are a number of reasons—ranging from heredity to environmental factors—that some become ill and others do not.

Infection, injury, and disease can all affect the sophisticated mechanisms of the ears, nose, and throat. Recognizing and understanding the various conditions and symptoms can help enormously when it comes to seeking treatment.

GENETIC AND HEREDITARY FACTORS

We all carry thousands of different genes, which give rise to the amazing diversity and variety of human beings. However, gene abnormalities may lead to a deformity that is immediately apparent at birth or may predispose an individual to a higher chance of developing an ENT condition later in life.

Problems at birth

A specific genetic abnormality may result in a condition known as microtia, where the the external framework of the ear, or pinna, is absent or malformed at birth.

MORE COMMON

MOTION SICKNESS	SINUSITIS
Up to 9 in 10 adults suffer from motion sickness at some time.	Approximately 32 million people have chronic sinusitis.
TINNITUS	HEARING LOSS
More than 44 million people in the United States suffer from tinnitus. This is 16 percent of the population.	More than 24 million people in the United States have significant hearing loss, 40 percent of whom are under 65 years old.

Babies with microtia are more likely to have other developmental problems in their middle and inner ears that affect their ability to hear. This may only become obvious as a child grows and starts interacting with others. Microtia is treatable: The malformed ear can be removed and a new one created from cartilage.

Some babies are predisposed to develop red vascular swellings beneath the skin called hemangiomas. When these occur in the airway, they may obstruct breathing, which can be fatal. Airway hemangiomas do not typically become enlarged until several weeks after birth, when

Average incidence of ENT problems
A variety of factors influence the long-term health of your ears, nose, and throat. The figures above show the number of people likely to contract an infection or other ENT problem in any given year.

they must be removed immediately. Newborn babies may also be predominantly nose rather than mouth breathers. Narrowing at the back of the nose, known as choanal atresia, may keep them from breathing effectively, leading to respiratory distress, although this can be detected and treated easily.

Problems in later life
Certain genes may make an individual more likely to develop particular types of cancer later in life, such as thyroid gland tumors. There may be no warning of the impending development of such a condition, although genetic testing of "high-risk" individuals enables doctors to spot a problem early so that steps can be taken to reduce any other risk factors that may contribute.

loud noise

ENVIRONMENTAL FACTORS
Although genetic factors may predispose an individual to the development of a particular disease, environmental factors act throughout life to influence whether or not a condition will

infection

develop. Reducing or avoiding some of these environmental factors can often help improve the chances of not developing an illness later in life.

Allergies
Many people are allergic to substances present in the atmosphere and in the home. These substances, which include pollen, dust mites, and animal dander (flakes of

Most ENT operations can now be performed on an outpatient basis. Only about 200,000 inpatient procedures were performed in the United States in 2000.

dead skin), are known as allergens. Exposure to allergens can cause nasal congestion, sneezing, and a runny nose. When reactions are triggered by tree or grass pollen during summer, the condition is known as hay fever. Treatment is based on avoidance of the allergen, together with drugs to relieve symptoms (see page 118).

Pollution
Atmospheric pollution can cause nasal congestion and rhinitis—inflammation of the nose's lining. Prolonged or highly concentrated exposure to specific occupational substances, such as nickel and hardwood shavings, is suspected of being linked to cancer of the sinuses.

Noise pollution
Noise is another form of damaging pollution. People who are regularly exposed to extreme levels of noise can suffer damage to the cochlea or labyrinth of the ear, leading to premature hearing loss.

LESS COMMON

SORE THROAT
Sore throats account for 2.1 percent of doctor visits, second only to coughs.

HAY FEVER
In 1997, 9 percent of adults were found to have hay fever.

OTITIS MEDIA
This is most common in children, affecting 75 percent by their third birthday.

MULTIPLE ENDOCRINE NEOPLASIA TYPE-1 (MEN1)
Affects fewer than 3–20 people per 100,000. Both genders and all races are affected equally.

ENT INFECTIONS
Infections are one of the most common reasons for visiting the doctor, and they can affect nearly every part of the head and neck.
- **Common ear infections** include otitis media (inflammation of the middle ear) and otitis externa (inflammation of the outer ear canal).
- **Common nose infections** include rhinitis and sinusitis.
- **Common throat infections** include pharyngitis (inflammation of the throat), tonsillitis, and glandular fever.

- **Common infections of the airways** include laryngitis (inflammation of the voice box) and, less commonly, tracheitis (inflammation of the windpipe).

Most of these conditions are acute, meaning that they are sudden, self-limited events, after which the patient returns to good health. Chronic infections are longer term chronic conditions that can last weeks, months, or years. Environmental factors such as damp living conditions, smoking, and heavy alcohol consumption can aggravate chronic infections.

TUMORS

These can affect the ears, nose, throat, and other parts of the head and neck. Tumors can be benign—that is, slow growing and confined to one area of the body—or malignant, more aggressive, faster growing, and more likely to spread to other areas. Cancers may occur in the sinuses, thyroid gland, salivary glands, throat, tongue, and larynx (voice box). A large number of tumors, particularly those affecting the inner lining of the nose, mouth, throat, and airways, are strongly linked to smoking. Avoiding the carcinogens in tobacco greatly reduces the chance of developing these tumors.

Tumors affecting the ear, nose, and throat can also appear on the skin of the head, face, neck, and ears and are commonly caused by exposure to strong sunlight.

Laser-activated cancer therapy for a tumor in the throat
A low-power red argon laser passes through four optical fiber wave-guides to kill cancer cells in a patient's throat by activating a drug (hematoporphyrin derivative) previously injected into the tumor. This procedure is still considered experimental in the United States.

These include malignant melanomas (tumors of the melanocytes, the cells that produce the skin's pigmentation) and basal cell carcinomas.

PHYSICAL INJURIES

Trauma, or physical injury, is a leading cause of illness and disability, particularly in young people. Common ear injuries include a perforated eardrum and the forming of a blood clot in the ear's external cartilage. The nose may bleed if picked frequently or punched; bleeding often stops with simple pressure and ice, but is likely to persist if a larger blood vessel has been severed. Foreign bodies such as pen caps, marbles, or cotton swabs can injure the ears, nose, or throat if inserted, inhaled, or swallowed. Other injuries can occur during surgery; for example, vocal fold paralysis might result from damage to a laryngeal nerve during a tricky thyroidectomy.

DRUGS

Side effects of several common drugs result in problems in the ears, nose, or throat. The antibiotic gentamicin, for example—often used intravenously to fight bloodstream infections—can cause profound deafness, particularly in genetically susceptible individuals. Some drugs used in the treatment of leukemias can affect balance and hearing. The loss is not necessarily related to the dose or duration of treatment with the drug; in some cases, it occurs after one dose but can cause permanent dizziness or deafness.

LIFESTYLE

Smoking is probably the greatest single influence on whether an individual develops certain illnesses or not. Excessive alcohol consumption is also detrimental to good health and has been linked to cancer of the mouth and tongue, especially in smokers. Although a direct link between dietary factors and the development of tumors has not been proven, experts believe that a balanced, low-fat diet with plenty of fruits and vegetables helps you maintain a healthy immune system capable of fighting off infection and recovering from injury.

AGING

The aging process is responsible for a number of gradual changes that result in progressive deterioration in the functioning of some body systems. Perhaps the most common example is hearing loss. Others include increased susceptibility to infections and certain types of tumors.

Meet the ENT specialists

Patients with problems relating to the ears, nose, and throat are usually referred to an ENT office. Here they will meet a wide range of specialists and technicians, who are trained to diagnose and treat all conditions of the neck and head.

The technically correct title for the surgical speciality of ENT is otolaryngology. This term encompasses conditions of the ears, nose, and throat, plus diseases of the base of the skull, head and neck, face, and trachea (windpipe). Treatment can involve the use of powerful operating microscopes, fiberoptic and rigid endoscopes, and lasers. The breadth of surgical skill required to meet the medical needs of patients necessitates close collaboration between ENT specialists and many other specialists, such as anesthesia staff, neurosurgeons (who specialize in the surgical treatment of the brain and spinal cord), plastic surgeons, and cardiothoracic surgeons (who specialize in the treatment of the heart and lungs).

ENT NURSE

The role of the ENT nurse is to provide care for post-operative ENT patients on hospital wards. They are trained to manage and care for patients with the full range of ENT conditions. Some nurses specialize in a particular aspect of patient care. For example, tracheotomy nurse specialists are now commonplace in larger ENT units; they offer expert advice on tracheostomies and are often the first port of call for tracheostomy patients who encounter problems at home.

AUDIOLOGICAL TECHNICIAN

Many patients visiting the ENT office need hearing tests. These are performed by audiological technicians who also prescribe and fit hearing aids, teach people how to use them effectively, and offer advice on other equipment and strategies that will help people deal with hearing loss. In addition, audiological technicians assess the functioning of the balance systems (see page 109).

SPEECH THERAPIST

Speech and language therapists are highly trained specialists who play a major role in treating patients with voice and speech problems and in the assessment and treatment of patients with swallowing difficulties (see page 131). Patients range from children who need a little

OTOLARYNGOLOGIST

The otolaryngologist treats ENT conditions and diseases, and many also now have subspecialties in one of these three areas, as well as in treating allergies or in performing surgery. Facial plastic surgery is another subspecialty. In the U.S., most facial cosmetic procedures are performed by otolaryngologists. All patients who visit an ENT office, or are admitted for an ENT procedure, are under the care of the consultant otolaryngologist.

remedial help with speech production to adults who have had their larynxes removed and require extensive support to regain effective communication skills (see page 130). In such cases, the speech therapist helps to decide which method of reestablishing speech will be most appropriate and then guides the patient in ways of overcoming the various voice and speech-related difficulties experienced after surgery, until rehabilitation is as complete as is possible in the circumstances.

SPECIALIST SURGEONS

Many ENT surgeons are now specializing in narrower fields of expertise. These subspecialties include
- otology—ear surgery
- skull base surgery
- rhinology—surgery on the nose and sinuses
- laryngology—voice and airway surgery
- head and neck surgery
- pediatric otolaryngology—ENT treatment for children.
Specialist head and neck surgeons, who are fully trained in ENT, now usually manage the majority of cases of head and neck tumors.

FINDING OUT WHAT IS WRONG

Diagnosis is the first step toward treatment and recovery from a problem, and the ENT office offers a whole range of investigative procedures designed to find out exactly what is wrong and why. Technological advances and modern teaching methods enable the specialists to analyze and treat problems—from a simple ear infection to a tumor—more quickly and effectively than ever before.

Medical history and examination

Doctors need to know as much as possible about a patient's medical history and current problems to determine the right treatment. At the consultation, the patient can describe symptoms and discuss any concerns.

LOOKING AT SYMPTOMS

Symptoms of many different conditions can affect your ears, nose, and throat, and your doctor will need to know all about your symptoms to reach an accurate diagnosis, so be sure to mention everything, even if you are not sure if it is relevant.

Ear pain and hearing problems

Otalgia, the medical term for earaches, can occur on the external part of the ear or deeper inside. However, earaches do not necessarily indicate that the problem originates in the ear. Some of the nerves that supply the ear also supply other regions, such as the throat and sinuses, and a problem in these areas may cause "referred" pain in the ears. A doctor who suspects that pain in an ear is referred will examine the mouth, nose, and sinuses, as well as the ear itself.

Swimming and ear infections
Swimming does not cause middle ear infections, although diving can be a contributing factor. Swimming in polluted water, however, may cause an outer ear infection.

Deafness or hearing loss can occur suddenly or gradually and can affect one or both ears. Hearing loss in children is a particular concern, because learning can suffer unless the cause is identified and treated promptly.

Tinnitus is the sensation of ringing or buzzing noise in the ear that only the sufferer can hear. A precise description of the noise is important, because tinnitus may be a feature of several different conditions (see page 152).

Common causes of ear infections

The two basic types of ear infection are otitis externa, or outer ear infection, and otitis media, middle ear infection.

• **Otitis media** occurs when the eustachian tube becomes blocked. When this happens, bacteria, which can normally drain freely back into the nose and throat to be harmlessly swallowed, become trapped in the mucus in the tube and start to multiply. If the tiny hair cells are damaged, by a cold virus for example, the mucus cannot get rid of the bacteria. The tube most often becomes blocked because of an infection, irritants such as cigarette smoke, or an allergy. Any of these may produce swelling and increase the amount of mucus produced in an attempt to get rid of the invaders. The same agents that block the eustachian tube also enlarge the glands at its opening, in effect closing its outlet. The mucus and saliva produced by teething babies can also cause the eustachian tube to function poorly. Increases in air pressure—in a plane, for example—can flatten the tube, effectively blocking it.

• **Otitis externa** is caused by bacteria entering the ear canal. This can happen to anyone who swims in polluted water, for example. People who pick at or play with their ears also run the risk of introducing bacteria into the ear.

Other ear-related problems

Fluid leaking from the ear may indicate a range of conditions. Pus signifies an infection, blood indicates an injury, and clear fluid may represent leakage of cerebrospinal fluid. The vast majority of cases of cerebrospinal fluid leakage result from trauma and, if identified and treated quickly with antibiotics and bed rest, get better without the need for surgery.

HELP YOUR DOCTOR HELP YOU

Your symptoms and lifestyle

If you are referred by your doctor to an ENT office, you will need to provide the specialists with as much information as possible. Making notes before your appointment on the following factors will make the consultation more useful.

• *Details of any past medical conditions: These help to put the current condition into context and help in its assessment and diagnosis. For example, a patient who has diabetes is more likely to suffer from recurrent and severe ear infections.*

• *The drug or treatment history of the current condition: This can be crucial. Knowledge that a patient with bleeding from the nose is taking the anticoagulant drug coumadin, for example, is of immense importance.*

• *Your family medical history: This gives doctors an indication of any illnesses that run in the family.*

• *Your job and lifestyle. Whether you work in an office or outdoors can be important, as can whether you swim, fly, or dive as a hobby. Be honest about whether you drink alcohol or smoke, and how much, because this can provide useful additional information.*

Health checks
A hearing test is part of your baby's developmental check at between six and nine months. The health provider will shake a rattle while your baby is distracted to check the response to a sound stimulus.

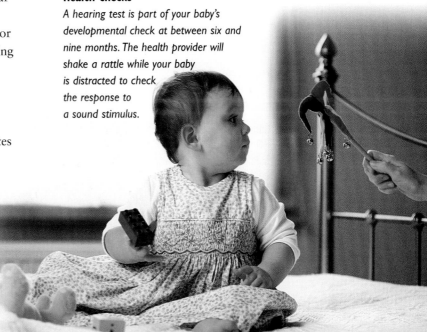

Dizziness is a vague term, so the doctor has to establish more precisely what kind of symptoms the patient is experiencing in order to diagnose the problem. Patients may feel that they or their surroundings are constantly moving or swirling around. This is known as vertigo and is caused by a problem in the vestibular part of the inner ear. Less severe symptoms involving lightheadedness, giddiness, or disorientation are rarely due to problems originating in the inner ear. The duration of a dizzy feeling is important, too: Dizziness lasting more than 24 hours may be caused by a viral infection of the vestibular system, whereas dizziness of much shorter duration is more likely to be due to Meniere's disease (see page 140).

A feeling of fullness in the ear is usually due to wax buildup, but it may indicate fluid in the middle ear.

The nose

A runny nose, sometimes accompanied by sneezing, usually indicates inflammation of the lining of the nose, or rhinitis. Patients with rhinitis may have a stuffy nose, but this is more common in those who have a deviated nasal septum or obstruction such as nasal polyps or a tumor.

Bleeding from the nose—often an alarming symptom—usually stops easily with simple pressure and ice. Bleeding is rarely a cause for concern, but when it recurs and is from one nostril only, it may be cause for investigation, because it may be a sign of a tumor.

Why are my ears so often blocked with wax?

Everybody's ears produce wax. In most cases, the small amounts made every day are naturally expelled from the ear, so the ears can be thought of as having their own "self-cleaning" mechanism. However, there are many reasons why some people's ears seem to build up, rather than get rid of, wax. There may be an excessive amount of wax produced (often an inherited problem), or the ear canals may be unusually narrow, making the "self-cleaning" process difficult. But by far the most common reason is the use of cotton swabs to clean the ears: These can push more wax into the ears than they remove. Cotton swabs can also damage the delicate skin of the ear canal. Common wisdom states that you should never put anything in your ear that is smaller than your elbow.

ASK THE EXPERT

The sinuses

Facial pain occurring between the eyes, on the side of the nose, or in the forehead may be an indication of inflammation and obstruction of the sinuses. Patients who have a sinus infection may also complain of a poor sense of smell.

EXTERNAL EAR   MIDDLE EAR   INTERNAL EAR (COCHLEA)   COCHLEAR NERVE AND CNS CONNECTIONS

——— CONDUCTIVE HEARING LOSS ———   ——— SENSORINEURAL HEARING LOSS ———

Otosclerosis or immobile ossicles

Wax buildup, inflammation, foreign bodies

Stapes fixation by otosclerosis

Nerve damage or tumors of the acoustic nerve

Perforation

Otitis media (glue ear, or fluid in the ear)

Sensory hearing loss, mumps, noise

Types of hearing loss

Hearing problems caused by injury to or blockage of the ear are called conductive if they occur between the external ear and the stapes bone; those from the stapes into the inner ear are called sensorineural. Different conditions cause problems in different areas.

The throat

Discomfort in the throat is usually a vague symptom, difficult to pinpoint to one specific area. It is most often caused by infection either in the lining of the throat (pharyngitis) or tonsils (tonsillitis). A lump in the throat is common and rarely points to serious underlying disease. It is often stress-related, but anyone who has difficulty in swallowing, or an earache as well, needs further investigation.

The airway

Hoarseness is not unusual in patients who have colds or in people who overuse their voices on a regular basis, such as singers or teachers. Overuse of the voice can trigger the growth of nodules or polyps on the vocal cords within the larynx (voice box); these benign growths generally make the voice sound hoarse. Occasionally, the cause of a hoarse voice turns out to be a tumor on the cords.

Stridor is the term used to describe a harsh sound produced typically on breathing in, but it can also occur on breathing out. It indicates narrowing of the larynx or trachea, possibly caused by a partial obstruction.

EXAMINING THE EAR

Doctors begin ear examinations with a close look at the outer part of the ear (the pinna), where a number of problems can be identified. Some injuries result in a blood clot beneath the skin of the ear. This is known as auricular hematoma. An abscess may develop either in a previously formed blood clot or on its own. A blood clot or abscess can destroy the cartilage of the outer ear. If this is left untreated, it may eventually lead to scarring, resulting in "cauliflower ear." Treatment involves the removal of the clot and drainage of the abscess.

Basal and squamous cell cancers—related to sun exposure —are also common on the outer ear but can be effectively treated using photodynamic therapy, surgery, or cryotherapy (freezing the skin).

Using an otoscope

External examination is followed by inspection of the ear canal and eardrum with an otoscope. This provides the doctor with a view of the ear canal and of the middle ear through the semitransparent eardrum. If ear wax blocks the view, the doctor removes the wax first. The otoscope enables the doctor to diagnose a range of ear problems such as eczema of the ear canal, which can become infected, particularly if the ear is not dried after swimming or showering. It is also possible to see boils or abscesses.

The view through an otoscope

a To examine the ear using an otoscope, the doctor gently pulls on the outer ear in order to straighten the ear canal to get a better view along it. The instrument is not inserted deeply: The light on its end enables the doctor to see to the eardrum and beyond.

b In a case of otitis media, a doctor would see redness and bulging of the eardrum caused by fluid buildup behind it.

c In persistent cases of otitis media, the eardrum may appear dull, and there might be fewer blood vessels than normal on its surface.

The appearance of the eardrum may give a clue as to the state of health of the middle ear. For example, fluid in the middle ear may cause bulging of the eardrum, and alter its surface color and degree of transparency. Perforations or infections may also affect the eardrum. It is also possible to see the ossicles through the eardrum. In patients who have had previous surgery or recurrent chronic infections, the ossicles may have eroded or be missing altogether, which can be a cause of hearing loss.

Using a microscope

For a more detailed look at the middle ear, the doctor will use a microscope, which magnifies the ear canal and eardrum. The use of a microscope also enables simple procedures to be carried out in the ENT office, including the removal of excessive wax or foreign bodies.

Examining the eustachian tubes

It is difficult for doctors to determine how well the eustachian tubes are working by otoscopic examination, but they can get an indication by checking the appearance of the eardrums. Patients with poor eustachian tube function are unable to force air into the tubes by simply pinching the nose and breathing out. This creates a negative pressure within the middle ear that can "suck in" the eardrum, drawing it away from the canal, and this can be seen with an otoscope. It does not prove that there is a problem with the eustachian tubes, however, so further examination is necessary.

Inside the human head
This false-color image produced from an MRI scan of a cross section through the head shows the nose at top center, the maxillary sinuses in yellow, and the sphenoidal sinuses in orange.

Ear examination is usually supplemented by tests of hearing and balance (see pages 107–9).

EXAMINING THE NOSE AND SINUSES

An examination of the nose starts with the doctor looking at its external appearance and shape. If there is a deformity, was it present at birth or due to an injury? The specialist must make this distinction because trauma-related deformities may be associated with injuries in other parts of the face not otherwise immediately apparent, such as fractures of the lower rim of the eye socket or damage to the teeth. Doctors also take a look at the overall symmetry of the face. Swelling or tenderness or both can indicate possible sinus infection.

EXPERIENCING AN ENDOSCOPE NASAL EXAMINATION

I had been feeling as if my nose was blocked on and off for some months. My doctor referred me to an ENT office, where the doctor examined my nose using a telescope.

Before the endoscope was inserted, the doctor sprayed my nostrils with a decongestant and anesthetic, which he told me was derived from cocaine. Over a period of about five minutes this relaxed my nostrils (which I wasn't really conscious of). He then started to insert the rigid endoscope.

I was conscious of the instrument being in my nose but there was no pain or even discomfort. The doctor moved the endoscope up into one nostril and maneuvered it into my nasal cavity. He then removed it and inserted it into my other nostril. He told me that he had found a polyp in my left nostril. The whole examination, including the wait for the anesthetic to take effect, took only 15 minutes.

Looking inside the nose

To begin, a doctor uses a speculum to hold the nostrils open and shines a light inside to look at the front of the nasal cavity. The back of the nose can be viewed using an angled mirror placed inside the mouth. The central part of the nose, however, can only be properly examined with a fiberoptic endoscope—flexible or rigid. A flexible endoscope is generally used for examining the throat, larynx, and back of the nose. Rigid endoscopes are used mainly to examine the nose and the sinuses.

Some patients who have had sinus surgery have large, open sinus cavities that are easily visible. In general, however, a doctor can't get a complete view of normal sinuses by examining the nose with a nasal speculum or an angled rigid endoscope. Instead, the patient is sent to an ENT office for further investigations, such as imaging tests.

EXAMINING THE THROAT

This investigation begins with a look at the patient's neck, which is best examined by palpation (gentle feeling) of the main structures. The key structures that concern an ENT

HAVING AN INDIRECT LARYNGOSCOPY

My doctor was unable to tell why my voice was so hoarse when I didn't have a sore throat or a cold, so he referred me to the local ENT office for a specialist examination of my larynx and vocal cords by indirect laryngoscopy.

The specialist at the clinic explained that he was going to position a special angled mirror in my mouth to obtain as good a view as possible of my larynx and vocal cords. Just before the examination began, he heated the mirror very slightly so that it wouldn't steam up when I breathed

on it. He asked me to concentrate on breathing through my mouth as normally as possible all through the examination.

I was asked to open my mouth and stick out my tongue, which the doctor gently grasped and pulled forward with a gauze swab. He then put the mirror into my mouth and positioned it so that it was touching the soft palate on the roof of my mouth, just in front of the uvula. Luckily I was able to stay relaxed and not gag. The doctor asked me to say a prolonged "e" so that my epiglottis would rise and he could see

into my larynx. Before I began to feel too uncomfortable, the doctor withdrew the mirror, explaining that he would replace it after I'd had a short rest. After several short examinations, the doctor said the test was over.

specialist are the lymph glands, which can easily be felt where they sit on either side of the Adam's apple, close to the major blood vessels. Lymph glands may be affected by tumors that originate in the mucosal lining of the throat, the base of the tongue, the nasopharynx (back of the nose), or the larynx.

Other structures in the neck that can require assessment include the thyroid gland. Because this is in the lower part of the neck, it is not easy to feel in most people. If the specialist can easily feel the thyroid gland, it is probably enlarged because of an autoimmune disorder such as Graves disease, or to a tumor, which needs further investigation.

Looking inside the mouth

The oral cavity—the tongue, tonsils, back wall of the throat, and lining of the mouth—is easily examined using a good light and two strong tongue depressors. The parotid salivary gland, in front of the ear, drains saliva into the mouth opposite the upper second molar, and this point in the mouth is marked by a prominent protrusion, which is easy to see. In addition, the floor of the mouth contains the salivary glands that drain saliva into the mouth. There may be cysts or swellings in these areas.

Examining the larynx is more difficult. It can be done in the ENT office either with a flexible endoscope, or by a technique known as "indirect laryngoscopy."

Indirect laryngoscopy

During an indirect laryngoscopy, the doctor puts an angled mirror on the end of a long metal rod into the mouth and uses it to examine the epiglottis, tongue base, and interior of the larynx, and—when necessary—the upper part of the trachea. The vocal cords can be seen and their movement assessed—if a vocal cord is paralyzed, it will not move when the patient talks or sings, as requested by the doctor.

One problem with indirect laryngoscopy is that some patients have a strong gag reflex and cannot tolerate a mirror pushed toward their throat. Local anesthetic spray can sometimes suppress this reflex so that the doctor can proceed with the examination. If this does not work, however, a specialist must use a flexible fiberoptic nasoendoscope, which is passed up one of the nostrils and through the nasal passages behind (see page 111).

Direct laryngoscopy

Sometimes the doctor wants to examine the internal structures of the larynx in more detail, perhaps to take biopsies of abnormal-looking tissue. This is done with the patient under a general anesthetic in the operating room, where the specialist has access to a range of rigid endoscopes. This examination of the larynx is known as direct (as opposed to indirect) laryngoscopy.

Videostroboscopy

This is the latest way of viewing and recording the vocal cords. A stroboscope is fed down the throat and into the larynx, where the cords are filmed in action, in a process called videostroboscopy.

Tighter
The vocal cords narrow as the patient vocalizes a sustained vowel.

What is it used for?

The movements of the vocal cords are complex and so the focus of much research. The creation of sound is no longer thought to be a simple case of the two vocal cords moving in and out against each other during speech. Each vocal cord is covered by a thin sheet of highly specialized mucosa that moves in a fluid manner by means of a series of rapid oscillations. This oscillatory movement is at a rate faster than the eye can detect: The only way to view the mucosal wave is via a videostroboscopy. This allows earlier detection of growths, scarring, broken blood vessels, and all kinds of abnormalities and malfunctioning than was previously possible.

How does it work?

The examination involves the use of a stroboscope—a flexible endoscope with a tiny camera and strobe light. Light is directed down the scope at a rate that effectively "freeze frames" the moving mucosal wave at a slightly different phase each time. The wave is seen to advance slowly, step by step, and any abnormalities in the construction of the wave can be more easily detected. The camera records the images and projects them, frame by frame, onto a TV monitor. Filming is in real time, but the specialist will later play back sequences in slow motion or examine images as a series of still photos. The patient is awake throughout and is usually asked to vocalize various sounds so the vocal cords can be filmed in action.

VIDEOSTROBOSCOPY IN ACTION

The vocal cords viewed through a stroboscope, as they appear on a television monitor. The cords are two bands of muscle, flanked by the ventricular folds.

Taut
The vocal cords are pulled taut as the patient intones a prolonged "eeee" followed by a prolonged "aaah."

Breathing out
As the patient breathes out, the vocal cords relax and open to allow air to be exhaled from the lungs.

Breathing in
The cords also open when the patient breathes in, so that air can pass down the larynx, into the trachea, and to the lungs.

Taking a deep breath
The vocal cords are wide open as the patient takes a deep breath.

Hearing tests

The many different hearing tests available at an ENT office range from simple whispering to the use of a computerized probe. They are designed to assess whether a patient's hearing is impaired, and, if so, to what degree and to discover what is causing the problem.

WHISPER TESTS

A specialist can gain a rough idea as to the level of hearing by conducting some simple "whisper" tests, whereby a number or a short word is whispered into each ear at varying distances. This is only a crude test and will need verification by a formal hearing assessment.

TUNING FORK TESTS

The Rinne and Weber tests, performed in sequence, assess the type and extent of hearing loss. They use a standard tuning fork with a resonant frequency of 512 hertz. A higher resonance might not be heard easily; anything lower might be felt as well as heard, confusing the test's result.

How do they work?

- The Rinne test is aimed at finding out how well a patient hears a sound transmitted to the middle and inner ear by air conduction (AC) in comparison with the same sound transmitted by bone conduction (BC) through vibration of the bony skull that vibrates the inner ear.
- The Weber test will detect whether a tuning fork placed at a midpoint between the ears is heard predominantly in just one ear.

What can they tell us?

Patients whose hearing is within the normal range hear AC better than BC and detect the tuning fork in the Weber test equally well with both ears.

Patients whose hearing loss is due to a problem with the conductive mechanisms of the middle ear should hear BC better than AC, because of a reduction in sound transmission by AC. These patients will hear the tuning fork in the Weber test more clearly in the ear with the conductive abnormality.

Patients whose hearing loss is caused by a problem with the neural connections to the brain—where the mechanisms transmitting sound to the inner ear are intact—will hear AC better than BC, because both will be reduced in proportion to each other. But the tuning fork in the Weber test will be heard best in the better hearing ear, rather than the ear where hearing is more impaired.

Rinne test

a A tuning fork is struck and then placed next to one ear. If the patient hears the sound, it is being transmitted by air conduction (AC). While the tuning fork is still resonating, its base is placed against the mastoid process (the bony protrusion behind the ear). If the patient hears the sound this time, it is being transmitted by bone conduction (BC). The process is repeated for the other ear.

Weber test

b The tuning fork is struck and then placed either in the middle of the forehead or on the vertex (highest point) of the head, in line with the center of the nose. The specialist records whether the patient hears the sound, and if so, whether it is heard equally well in both ears or mainly in one ear or the other.

AUDIOMETRY

An audiometry test is carried out at an ENT office in a soundproof room. The test is designed to measure air conduction (AC) and bone conduction (BC) thresholds.

How does it work?

To test for AC thresholds, the patient wears headphones so that the only sound that can be heard is that produced by the audiometer—the hearing test machine. Common practice is to test hearing at distinct set frequencies only, usually 250 or 500 hertz, or 1, 2, 4, and 8 kilohertz. At each frequency, a sound is played to each ear in turn, and the patient must press a button to indicate that he or she heard the sound. The loudness or intensity of the sound is gradually decreased until the patient does not respond. The quietest sound at which the patient registers a response is called the threshold for that particular frequency. This is repeated for the remaining frequencies and then for the other ear.

The technician makes a graph to show the hearing thresholds for each frequency. The level, or loudness, of sound is measured in decibels, or dB. This is a logarithmic scale, which means that a sound measured at 20 decibels has ten times the sound intensity of a sound of 10 decibels, not twice the intensity.

The audiological technician can test BC thresholds by applying a special bone vibrator to the mastoid process (the prominent bony protrusion behind the ear) and then following the same procedure. With both AC and BC tests completed, the specialist can then examine any differences in the AC and BC thresholds.

Audiometric hearing test
The audiological technician sends sounds of varying volume through the earphones worn by the child, and the child presses a button whenever a sound is heard. To make the test more interesting, the sounds are associated with pictures on a television monitor.

TYMPANOMETRY

This hearing test helps the ENT specialist assess the functioning of the eustachian tubes, and—if there is an abnormality—whether treatment is necessary or possible.

How does it work?

The audiologist inserts a probe into the outer part of the patient's ear canal. The probe calculates the eardrum's movement at different pressures produced by the probe and thereby gains an impression of the pressure within the middle ear. Maximum movement of the drum occurs when pressure produced by the probe in the canal is equal to pressure within the middle ear. A computer attached to the probe produces a graph to show the test results.

Tympanogram

The test measures the level of mobility (compliance) of ossicles within the middle ear with varying air pressures. Low mobility means that the eardrum and ossicles are stiff or obstructed; the likely cause is fluid in the middle ear. High mobility shows that the drum is too flaccid and may indicate damage.

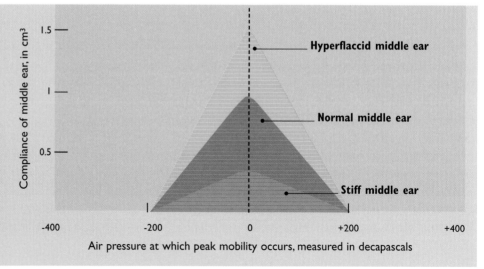

Compliance of middle ear, in cm³

1.5

1

0.5

-400   -200   0   +200   +400

Hyperflaccid middle ear

Normal middle ear

Stiff middle ear

Air pressure at which peak mobility occurs, measured in decapascals

Tests of balance

In addition to testing hearing, audiology departments also perform balance tests. ENT specialists may request one of these tests for a patient who is suffering from vertigo (severe dizziness) for which there is no obvious cause.

There are various balance tests, each one designed to assess a separate aspect of the balance mechanism. If results are to be accurate, it is vital that patients stop taking any sedatives designed to suppress disturbances of the inner ear at least 48 hours before a test takes place.

NYSTAGMUS: THE KEY TO BALANCE TESTING

If a patient experiences the dizziness known as vertigo, it is often due to an abnormality in the inner ear balance system in one ear or the other. The brain receives incorrect information from the abnormal side, which indicates that the body is spinning in one particular direction, and it therefore compensates by causing the eyes to undergo rapid, involuntary oscillatory movements toward the opposite side. These eye movements are called nystagmus.

ENT experts categorize nystagmus according to its direction (mainly to the left or right) or its degree, which is related to the severity of the inner ear abnormality. These parameters can be recorded by a technique known as electronystagmography (ENG), in which an audiological technician attaches electrodes to the skin close to the patient's eyes; the electrodes detect minute changes in the electrical potential generated by even the tiniest of eye movements.

CALORIC TESTS

Caloric testing is done to determine whether the patient has a diseased labyrinth (the fluid-filled system of coiled bony tubes that makes up the inner ear and, among other things, controls balance). Some people feel uncomfortable or even dizzy when cold or warm water is squirted into their ear. It is this phenomenon that forms the basis of the tests, in which water of two different temperatures—86°F and 111°F—is introduced into each ear in turn.

The resulting change of temperature within the inner ear triggers motion currents in the fluid contained within the labyrinth. This may give rise to a sensation of dizziness in the patient, followed by nystagmus. The degree of the nystagmus (measured by ENG) varies according to the severity of the patient's condition; the

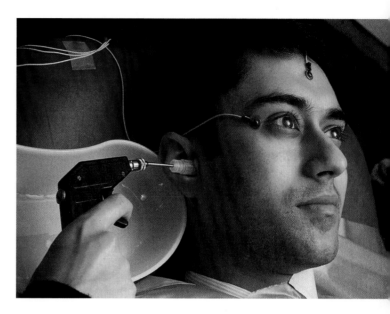

Caloric test in action
The electrodes attached to the patient's skin, above and next to his eyes, measure involuntary eye movement by electronystagmography (ENG). This indicates what degree of dizziness, if any, is being induced by the water being squirted into his ear.

direction varies according to the temperature of the water. If the labyrinth is healthy, nystagmus will occur for a predictable period. If there is a problem, nystagmus will occur for a short time, or not at all.

ROTATORY CHAIR TEST

This test stimulates nystagmus so that it can be measured accurately. A patient with a diseased inner ear becomes less dizzy than a person with healthy ears. The patient sits, with his or her eyes closed, in a swivel chair. The audiologist spins the chair around 10 times in a total time of 20 seconds and then brings the chair to an abrupt stop. This procedure will cause nystagmus in almost all patients, and the audiologist records the direction and degree manually or via ENG.

Care must be taken when performing a rotatory chair test, particularly with patients suffering from severe vertigo, because the stimulus is fairly significant and can make the condition worse.

Investigative tests of the nose

When doctors test the working of the nose, they are trying to establish the cause of a variety of problems and abnormalities. Tests fall into three main categories: allergy tests, tests to assess a patient's sense of smell, and tests of the behavior of the nasal hairs.

ALLERGY TESTS

Because such a large number of patients suffer from allergic rhinitis, it is hardly surprising that allergy tests are among the most common investigations to take place in the ENT office. They usually involve provoking and then observing a series of skin reactions to a variety of different allergens (substances that can provoke an allergic reaction), including grass pollen, house dust, dust mites, cat and dog hairs, feathers, and milk. The ENT nurse places a small quantity of protein prepared from each allergen onto a patient's forearm. If the patient is allergic to any of the substances, a reddish, slightly raised weal will appear.

The tests may not be valid if the patient is taking antihistamines, such as for hay fever, as these will reduce any allergic response to the test substances. In such circumstances, the nurse and doctor will probably decide to postpone the test until the patient has been free from the drug for a period of at least 48 hours.

TESTS ASSESSING THE SENSE OF SMELL

Olfactory tests—tests of the sense of smell—aim to evaluate the range of smells a patient can pick up and how well the odors are detected. The simplest olfactory test involves patient identification of a range of standard liquid odors. This crude test assumes that the patient is already familiar with all the smells being offered.

More accurate, although not common in the U.S., is electro-olfactography (EOG), in which an electrode is placed next to the olfactory nasal lining, high in the nasal cavity. The patient sniffs a succession of odors, and the electrode detects the electrical potential generated by the olfactory cells in response to each odor.

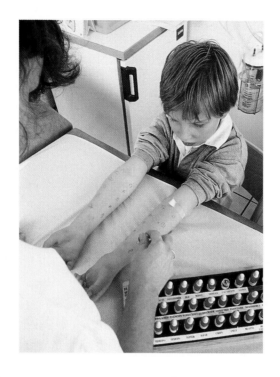

Testing for a reaction
This boy's arms are being painted with a variety of allergens to try to pinpoint which is causing his allergic rhinitis.

MUCOCILIARY FUNCTION TESTING

The nasal lining is covered by a layer of highly specialized cilia (tiny hairlike structures) that beat at a rate of approximately 15 times per second to move overlying mucus to the back of the nose so it can be swallowed. This is known as mucociliary clearance or transport. It can be measured by placing a drop of saccharin just inside the nose and asking the patient to swallow every 30 seconds. The time taken for the patient to experience a sweet taste should be 12 to 15 minutes if ciliary beat frequency is normal. If it takes longer than this, there is a problem with ciliary function.

Looking inside the nose and throat

Of all the methods used by ENT specialists to examine the interior of the nose, the pharynx and larynx, flexible nasopharyngoscopy is probably the most effective.

A nasopharyngoscopy is a test in which a doctor—generally an ENT specialist—uses a flexible fiberoptic nasoendoscope to examine a patient's upper airway. The doctor may be looking for problems or abnormalities in the nose, but the procedure is most commonly employed to make a detailed examination of the throat and larynx.

Fiberoptic cables within the nasoendoscope's narrow tubing transmits images from inside the patient's head and neck to the eye of the specialist via an optical system or a miniature video camera. If a video camera is used, the examination can be displayed on a monitor or recorded and played back later or both.

The specialist usually guides the tip of the nasoendoscope down the throat via the patient's nose. This is because introducing it through the mouth can trigger the gag reflex, which might make the patient jerk his or her head or even bite on the end of the scope.

A long and winding road
The doctor looks down the eyepiece of the nasoendoscope as he guides the instrument's tubing up through one of the patient's nostrils, along the nasal passages, and down the throat.

EXPERIENCING A FLEXIBLE NASOPHARYNGOSCOPY

My doctor thought a closer look at my throat and larynx was needed and so referred me to the ENT office for an examination with a flexible nasoendoscope.

The doctor sprayed one of my nostrils with a combined anesthetic and decongestant that took about three minutes to take effect. With the nostril completely numb, he gently guided the scope up my nose while looking through the eyepiece. When he was sure the scope had reached the back of my nose, he used the controls to angle it in a downward direction. The doctor guided it past the soft palate, the back wall of the pharynx, and the base of my tongue, so that he could see any abnormalities. Finally, it reached my larynx, at which point he asked me to sing the letter "e" so that he could assess the movements of my vocal cords.

Once the doctor was happy that he had seen all there was to see, he carefully removed the scope. Much to my relief, it hadn't turned out to be a painful process, although I had felt some discomfort.

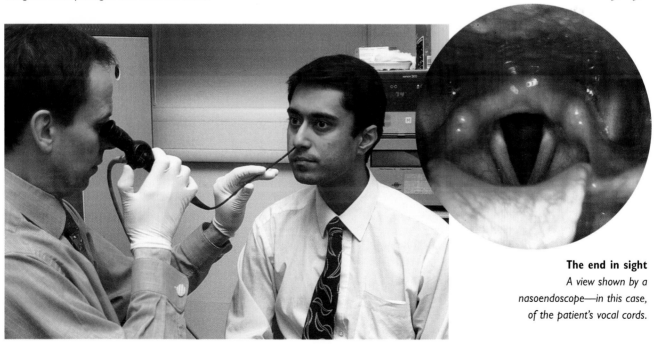

The end in sight
A view shown by a nasoendoscope—in this case, of the patient's vocal cords.

Investigating a lump in the neck

Swellings or lumps in the neck often cause patients great concern. In order to allay their fears, doctors refer a significant proportion to the ENT office for speedy diagnosis. The good news is that in most cases, the swellings are benign.

CAUSES FOR CONCERN

Features in the patient's history that may be cause for concern include a sudden, rapid enlargement in a swelling in the neck and the presence of deep, unrelenting pain that does not respond to simple painkillers. A breakdown in the skin overlying a lesion or symptoms from within the pharynx or other internal structure—such as a lump, difficulty swallowing, hoarseness of the voice, or earaches caused by referred pain—are also symptoms the doctor will want to investigate.

INITIAL INVESTIGATIONS

The specialist will carry out a thorough examination of the neck; look into the mouth, nose, and ears; and then perform a flexible nasoendoscopy in order to study all aspects of the pharynx and larynx. The investigative process continues with blood tests to establish the state of the patient's blood before treatment begins. The tests are used to tell whether the patient is anemic, what chemicals are dissolved in the plasma, and whether there are any traces of infection in the blood.

If a lung tumor is suspected, a chest X-ray follows. The X-ray is also used to check for any signs of a chest infection or potential heart failure, which may put the patient at risk if a general anesthetic becomes necessary at some future date.

In addition to these tests, the specialist selects the tests that are the most appropriate for each individual case.

BARIUM SWALLOW OR VIDEOFLUOROSCOPY

The specialist may recommend a barium swallow, particularly if difficulty in swallowing is a key symptom. In this procedure, the patient swallows a radiopaque barium-containing liquid that lines the pharynx and esophagus and shows up brightly when the radiologist takes X-ray pictures. This test highlights any lesion that is narrowing the pharynx or esophagus, which may have been out of range of the nasoendoscopic examination.

ASPIRATING A LUMP

Fine-needle aspiration cytology (FNAC) has revolutionized the assessment of patients with cancerous and benign neck swellings by allowing doctors to obtain samples of tissue without the patient having to undergo surgery. It is also used as an aid in the diagnosis of lumps in other parts of the body, including the breast. The test is carried out by an ENT specialist or by a cytopathologist (a specialist in the study of cells). A needle and syringe are used to draw out a sample of material from the lump. The needle is fine enough to avoid aspirating blood as well as cells. The material from the lump is sent to the laboratory for analysis at once, and the results of the test are often available just a few hours later.

Three common diagnostic tests

a and **b** Taking a blood sample

A technician examines a blood sample in a test tube. Highly magnified blood cells are taken from a patient with anemia (see inset). Because the red blood cells lack iron, an essential component of the blood pigment hemoglobin, they stain poorly. (Just two white blood cells are identifiable, both stained purple.) Anemia is a symptom, not a disease, so a specialist must now identify the disorder that is causing the anemia. There is a possibility that it could be cancer.

c and **d** A barium swallow

A patient stands ready to take a swallow from a glass of barium meal and follow its progress on the monitor attached to the digital X-ray system. The drink contains barium sulfate, a substance opaque to X-rays that outlines regions of the digestive tract. Here, the pharynx and esophagus are being checked for abnormalities such as a tumor. The colored X-ray shows the esophagus of a patient who is in the act of swallowing barium meal in red—the upper part of the esophagus appears narrow as muscles constrict to swallow the drink.

e Having a lump aspirated

The patient is undergoing a fine-needle aspiration cytology (FNAC) test as part of an investigation into a lump in her thyroid gland. The aim of the test is to remove a small quantity of cells from within the lump, and send them to the laboratory for immediate analysis. A local anesthetic can cause more discomfort afterward than the procedure itself, so the patient is not anesthetized. After cleaning the skin with a swab, the specialist inserts a needle attached to a syringe into the lump and, making several "passes," draws out the tissue needed, which is then smeared onto several glass slides and sent to the laboratory.

Normal and cancerous cells

These two cell samples—seen here stained and magnified—were removed by FNAC from tissue from two different patients. They demonstrate the striking difference between normal squamous cells (far right) and cancerous squamous cells (near right).

Cancers of the head and neck that are diagnosed while still small and localized have a cure rate of over 80 percent.

Microbiological testing

Many patients arrive at ENT clinics with an infection, such as an inflamed, painful ear or acute tonsillitis. Microbiological testing allows the organism responsible for the infection—the pathogen—to be identified, so that the most effective drugs can be prescribed.

TAKING A SAMPLE

The first stage is to take a sample of the infected area and send it to the laboratory for analysis. In the case of an infection of the external part of the ear canal, for example, it is easy enough to take a swab of the inflammatory discharge in the ear canal.

If the patient has an infection of the middle ear, the eardrum may be bulging, red, and inflamed, indicating that there is infected fluid, known as an effusion, in the middle ear. The pain can sometimes be so severe that it has to be relieved by making a tiny incision in the eardrum to release the fluid; when this happens, some of the fluid can be sent for analysis.

In the case of a neck abscess, a sample of the contents can be drawn out using a needle and syringe.

CULTURING THE SAMPLE

Once the sample has reached the laboratory, a microbiology technician distributes it evenly across the surface of a specialized agar jelly plate. The plate is then incubated in a warm environment for 48 hours. At the end of this period, the pathogens (the microorganisms causing the infection) in the sample will have multiplied, making analysis easier. In the case of hardier organisms an incubation period of up to six weeks is often necessary.

IDENTIFYING THE PATHOGEN

The microbiologist removes part of the colony of organisms and places it on a glass slide for examination under a microscope. Each organism has a unique appearance, enabling the microbiologist to make a precise identification. Viruses are so small that they cannot be examined using an ordinary light microscope, however.

Diphtheria bacterium
A rod-shaped diphtheria bacterium (shown here in cross section) lies on the surface of the throat. Treatment is with antitoxins and penicillin.

Instead, the microbiologist must use an electron microscope, which provides magnification a thousand times greater than a light microscope.

TAKING A COMPLETE BLOOD COUNT

A complete blood count (CBC) can help to establish the seriousness of the infection by telling the specialist the total white blood cell count of the patient. In the presence of an infection, the number of white cells will usually have increased. If a patient has leukemia, however, the number of white cells may actually have fallen, rather than increased, making it difficult for the patient to resist even the mildest infections.

***Streptococcus* bacteria**
These chains of Streptococcus pyogenes *bacteria are attached to a tonsil. They are surrounded by a layer of mucus (falsely colored blue).* Streptococcus pyogenes *can cause sore throats, tonsillitis, scarlet fever, and wound infections.*

Imaging techniques

The tools that enable doctors to visualize the structures inside the body that can't otherwise be seen—notably X-ray and scanning machines—are invaluable in the ENT office. These tools can locate tumors, establish the severity of conditions such as sinusitis, and even find foreign objects such as fish bones.

X-RAYS

In spite of newer developments in imaging techniques, X-rays are still a vital detecting tool for diseases and disorders of the ears, nose, and throat. For example, if a patient has accidentally swallowed a fish bone that may have lodged itself somewhere in the pharynx, an X-ray can help the specialist identify where the bone is. For patients with acute sinusitis, an X-ray of the sinuses will often help diagnose the severity of the condition. However, a patient with a fractured nose does not usually require an X-ray, because a doctor can diagnose a fractured nose by physical examination.

CT SCANNING

Computerized tomography (CT) scanning is particularly useful in ENT because many of the structures of the ears, nose, and throat can't be seen properly, even with the aid of nasoendoscopy. During a CT scan, a series of X-rays are directed at the specific area in question, from a variety of angles and planes. The points at which the X-ray beams intersect enable the scanner's computer to calculate precisely how much of the X-ray beam has been absorbed by the tissue. In this way, the computer produces a detailed picture of the target area, highlighting both normal structures and abnormal lesions.

CT scanning is used for examining the sinuses in more detail than an X-ray can provide, mapping out the lymph glands in the neck in cases of suspected cancer, and visualizing the middle ear and mastoid system for evidence of chronic infections.

MRI

Magnetic resonance imaging (MRI) employs magnets rather than X-rays to scan the body. The patient is asked to lie on a couch, which then slowly moves through what is in effect a long, hollow, cylindrical magnet. The magnet causes a realignment of the hydrogen atoms present within the cells of the area under investigation. When the hydrogen atoms assume their original state, there is a loss of energy. The MRI computer detects this

Images of the head
a A computerized tomography (CT) scan presents a profile of a human head, with bone shown as pink or blue, and soft tissue—including the nasal cavity and throat—colored yellow or green.
b Magnetic resonance imaging (MRI) techniques produced these cross sections through a human head, facing forward. The colored image clearly shows the nasal cavity, flanked on either side by the air-filled maxillary sinuses.

shift in energy and converts it into an electronic form. The sum total of all of the energy shifts is then compiled into a detailed image.

MRIs are mainly used in the ENT clinic to diagnose small tumors of the auditory nerve, swellings related to the salivary glands, and (occasionally) tumors of the sinuses.

Whereas CT scanning is especially good at imaging bony structures, MRI scanning's strength lies in detecting soft tissues including muscle, glands, and fat. The advantage of an MRI is that the patient avoids exposure to X-rays, but many patients find MRIs claustrophobic. Also, metallic implants in the body, such as artificial hips, heart valves, or pacemakers can interfere with the magnetic image, and the magnetic field can also interfere with the implants themselves. The radiologist makes the final decision as to whether it is safe to proceed with the scan.

CURRENT TREATMENTS

Many ear, nose, and throat problems can be resolved with the help of drugs; others need treatment in the form of surgery. Some surgical procedures are minor and can be performed as outpatient procedures under local anesthetic, whereas others—especially operations to restore hearing—require a stay in the hospital followed by rehabilitation. Whatever the patient's condition and treatment, staff at the ENT office are there to help, using cutting edge diagnostic and surgical equipment, coupled with specialist expertise.

Drug therapy

Today's advanced drugs are designed to target and treat a whole range of ear, nose, and throat conditions, from severe vertigo to the common cold.

Drugs can be administered either topically or systemically. Topical drugs are applied to the surface to be treated, for example the skin or nasal lining, and take the form of cream or ointment, drops, or spray. They deliver the drug to the targeted area and minimize its absorption into the bloodstream. Systemic drugs are swallowed or injected, after which they are absorbed into the bloodstream, which distributes them to the targeted areas of the body.

DRUGS FOR EAR CONDITIONS
Drugs for the external parts of the ear are usually given topically, generally in the form of drops. In cases of severe ear infection, discharge in the ear canal will need to be cleared by microsuction. If the ear canal is very swollen, the doctor will insert a small foam wick that soaks up the drops and allows them to reach the infected ear canal. The wick is left in place for a few days.
- **Drops for hardened wax in the ear** Wax can be softened by adding warm olive oil, a solution of baking soda and water, or one of the many proprietary eardrops available over the counter to the ear canal. One of these may be sufficient by itself to clear the wax; if not, the doctor can remove it by syringing or microsuction.

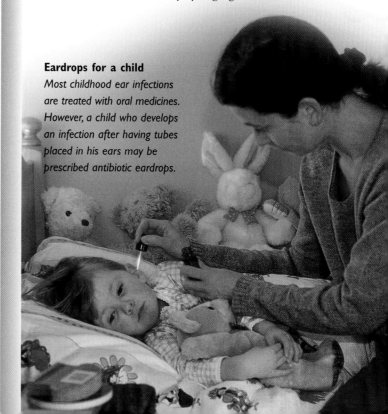

Eardrops for a child
Most childhood ear infections are treated with oral medicines. However, a child who develops an infection after having tubes placed in his ears may be prescribed antibiotic eardrops.

Irrigating an ear
The syringe squirts water upward so that it falls behind the blockage and forces the wax out of the ear. This must be performed by trained personnel using the correct equipment to avoid damage to the ear.

- **Antibiotic eardrops for the outer ear** An external ear inflammation (otitis externa) caused by bacterial infection is generally safely and effectively treated with antibiotic eardrops. Occasionally, the drops cause an allergic skin reaction. A combination of antibiotics and steroids (in drop form) will reduce this reaction and help to reduce swelling of the skin in the infected ear canal.
- **Antibiotics for the middle ear** Systemic antibiotics are generally needed for middle ear infections, which are particularly common in children. However, if there is a long-standing perforation of the eardrum, which divides the outer and middle ears, antibiotic drops can be extremely effective. There is a slight risk that some antibiotic drops could damage the tiny "hair cells" in the inner ear and thereby cause some loss of hearing and dizziness. To minimize this risk, antibiotic drops should be stopped as soon as the infection clears or if the patient experiences any problems with balance.
- **Antifungal eardrops** These are used to treat fungal external ear infections.
- **Acetic acid eardrops and sprays** These treat external ear infections by creating an acidic environment that restricts bacterial and fungal growth.
- **Steroid eardrops** Steroid drops are used to ease an allergic skin reaction that is not infected, such as eczema.

Is syringing the ears ever necessary, and can it be harmful?

Wax in the ears serves a useful protective role. Under normal circumstances, the ears are self-cleaning and it is not necessary to remove any wax. Occasionally, however, too much wax builds up. Impacted wax is a major cause of reversible hearing loss in the elderly.

Your doctor will recommend irrigation if wax is affecting your hearing, causing discomfort, or preventing an examination of the eardrum. Before irrigation, you will be asked to use eardrops to soften the wax: This may make irrigation easier. Doctors are reluctant to irrigate ears in patients with a history of ear disease or surgery. An inappropriately directed jet of water may force wax deeper into the ear or perforate the eardrum, so removal under a microscope is recommended. Irrigation has been thought to cause tinnitus, but the links are unproven; it may be that the beginnings of the tinnitus were present before irrigation took place, but it was assumed the irrigation was to blame.

ASK THE EXPERT

DRUGS FOR VERTIGO AND MOTION SICKNESS
Abnormalities of the vestibular (balance) system result in vertigo (dizziness), and this is often associated with nausea or vomiting or both, particularly during travel. These symptoms are treated with vestibular sedatives—drugs that act on the brain to suppress inappropriate signals from the inner ear but can also cause drowsiness.

- **Diphenhydrate and meclizine** These are medications that can be obtained over the counter.
- **Prochlorperazine** This is available as a sublingual (placed under the tongue but not swallowed) tablet or in suppository form. The suppository or sublingual forms are helpful if vomiting accompanies the dizziness.
- **Betahistine** Often prescribed to patients with recurrent symptoms. This medicine is intended for regular long-term use to prevent attacks rather than to treat acute symptoms of dizziness. This has not yet been approved by the FDA, so it is not available in the U.S. It is used in 70 countries.

Some people get motion sickness watching a movie on a large screen: The mismatch of signals to the ears, eyes, and brain triggers the condition.

DRUGS FOR RHINITIS AND SINUSITIS

The doctor's choice of drops or spray for the nose depends on the cause of the malady, which is generally manifested by rhinitis—inflammation of the nose's mucous membrane.

Allergies are a frequent cause of rhinitis and often contribute to conditions such as glue ear (fluid in the ear), asthma, and eczema. The first step in treatment is to identify and avoid the allergens that are causing a reaction.

- **Antihistamines** These can be taken topically or systemically. Available without prescription, tablets are very effective when taken for allergic rhinitis. Antihistamine sprays require a prescription and have to be used more frequently than steroid sprays, but many tablet forms are intended to be taken just once a day.
- **Nasal steroid sprays** These reduce the blockage, sneezing, and nasal discharge associated with rhinitis and are particularly effective if the rhinitis is allergic. It is best to take steroids topically to keep any side effects to a minimum. Doctors will also prescribe these medicines in combination with antibiotics to treat infective sinusitis.
- **Decongestants** These topical medicines work by constricting the blood vessels in the nasal lining, which helps decongest the nose. They are effective and safe if taken over a few days (no longer than a week) to treat a cold, sinusitis, or severe nasal allergies.
- **Cromolyn sodium** This antiallergy drug, available in spray form, does not contain steroids and is therefore often prescribed for children.

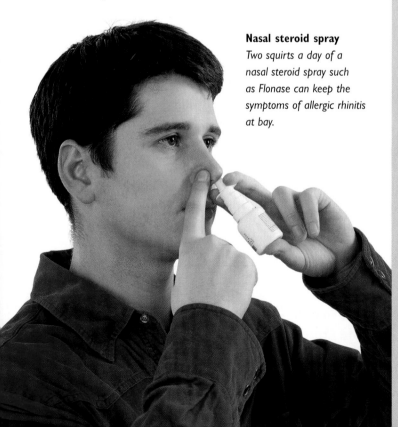

Nasal steroid spray
Two squirts a day of a nasal steroid spray such as Flonase can keep the symptoms of allergic rhinitis at bay.

Surgical solutions

Some ear, nose, and throat conditions need surgery, much of which is routine and—thanks to modern technology—safer than ever before. Procedures vary, and staff at the ENT office are there to discuss any concerns before and after the operation.

BEFORE AN OPERATION

The decision to have an operation is usually made by the patient and the ENT surgeon during an outpatient consultation. Concerns to discuss include the following:

- If the operation goes well, what are the expected benefits, and what are the chances of a successful long-term outcome?
- What if the operation goes badly? What are the possible complications?
- What is the likely outcome without the operation?

Of course, there are many other factors that will influence the decision to undergo an operation, including

- How long is the expected hospital stay?
- What is the expected recovery period? Will care be necessary at home after leaving hospital? When will it be possible to resume work?

The preadmission clinic

It may be difficult for the patient to remember all the necessary information with just one consultation, so many hospitals run a preadmission clinic, which the patient attends a few weeks before the operation. This allows medical staff to reassess the patient's condition prior to surgery and to complete routine admission tests. It also gives the patient an opportunity to go over the surgical process again and ask more questions.

SPECIAL REQUIREMENTS FOR ENT SURGERY

Many of the operations performed on the ear, nose, or throat are delicate procedures, undertaken on tiny structures and with limited access. All this presents the medical team with a special set of challenges.

Minimizing bleeding

When operating on tricky, delicate areas within the ears, nose, and throat, it is best to keep bleeding to an absolute minimum. Manipulation of the general anesthetic helps with this by maintaining blood pressure at a low, yet safe, level, so that bleeding is minimal.

Special equipment for microscopic surgery

The microscopic size of many structures within the ears, nose, and throat necessitates special equipment. The operating microscope and endoscope have dramatically improved the visualization of these areas and therefore the quality of surgery carried out. The microscope is routinely used in microlaryngeal (voice box) surgery and all middle ear and mastoid surgery. The endoscope is used in sinus surgery and for examination of the throat and trachea.

Keeping the airway open

Operations on the throat require close collaboration between the surgeon and anesthetist, so that the need for access for surgery does not threaten maintenance of the airway. Because general anesthesia relaxes the throat and chest muscles, the patient's breathing is supported by a tube placed in the throat. This tube maintains a safe passage for air through the throat and is designed in such a way that it prevents the passage of any foreign matter into the lungs.

On the cutting edge
Breakthroughs in surgical techniques and the quality of implants are arriving fast and furious in the world of ear, nose, and throat surgery.

ENDOSCOPIC SINUS SURGERY
The use of microscopes, endoscopes, and TV monitors has done much to overcome problems traditionally faced by a surgeon operating on the sinuses. The sinuses are very difficult to access, but their proximity to the eyes and brain demands that surgery must be performed with total precision.

INSERTING TUBES BY LASER
Instead of cutting into an eardrum with a scalpel before inserting an ear tube, the latest way is to use a laser. The laser both speeds up the operation and reduces the patient's discomfort, and so it allows the procedure to be performed under a local rather than a general anesthetic. This is not widely done in the United States.

TOTALLY IMPLANTED HEARING AIDS
A digital hearing aid fitted within the middle ear can deliver a quality of hearing unattainable by more conventional aids and yet can be invisible to the eye. There are still problems to be solved—especially how to maintain and repair a digital aid without surgery—but interest is so great that these difficulties will almost certainly be overcome.

NEW SPEECH FOR THE VOICELESS
Surgical implants are the way forward for patients who have lost their voice following removal of the larynx (voice box). A valve is implanted in the trachea (windpipe) that enables the patient to produce "speech" when breathing out.

Surgery on the ears

Surgeons perform a range of operations on the ears, the majority of which are to restore or improve impaired hearing. ENT specialists, however, may also carry out cosmetic surgery to improve the profile of the ears.

REMOVING A FOREIGN BODY

Foreign bodies of many different shapes and sizes can get stuck in the ear canal. When removing a foreign body, the doctor takes great care to avoid damaging the eardrum, ossicles (the small bones of the middle ear), or the inner ear. Such damage could lead to hearing loss, tinnitus, or vertigo. The foreign body is removed under direct vision, using an operating microscope—if necessary—and a hook, alligator forceps, or suction tube. In most cases involving adults, objects are removed without anesthetic in the outpatient clinic, but a child who will wriggle around may need a general anesthetic.

INSERTING EAR TUBES FOR GLUE EAR

Glue ear (fluid in the ear) is the popular name for a condition in which fluid produced by the lining of the middle ear collects behind the eardrum. It occurs most

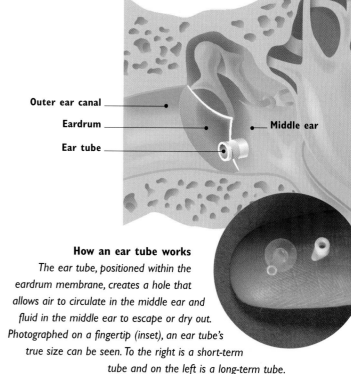

Outer ear canal

Eardrum

Ear tube

Middle ear

How an ear tube works
The ear tube, positioned within the eardrum membrane, creates a hole that allows air to circulate in the middle ear and fluid in the middle ear to escape or dry out. Photographed on a fingertip (inset), an ear tube's true size can be seen. To the right is a short-term tube and on the left is a long-term tube.

often in children, usually in both ears. The condition causes partial deafness; if it doesn't resolve, the specialist may carry out an operation called a myringotomy. In this procedure, the eardrum is cut with a microscopic scalpel so that the fluid can escape.

To prevent the incision from healing over and the glue ear from recurring, a plastic ventilation tube or ear tube is inserted into the incised eardrum. The operation can sometimes be performed under a local anesthetic, but most patients—especially children—require a general anesthetic. After insertion, the tubes can cause a mild infection. The resulting discharge is easily treated by cleaning the ear canal and applying antibiotic eardrops.

Short-term ear tubes are designed to be slowly and painlessly extruded by the eardrum—skin slowly collects under the rim of the tube and pushes the tube out. This takes place over 6–15 months, which is usually long enough for the condition to have resolved. In recurrent cases, doctors may use a nonextruding ventilation tube that is surgically removed 2–3 years later.

REPAIRING A PERFORATED EARDRUM

The eardrum is a thin and delicate structure. It can become perforated as a result of

- infection;
- direct trauma caused by the insertion of items such as cotton swabs; or
- indirect trauma, such as a bomb blast or barotrauma from rapid ascent or descent when flying or diving.

Perforations usually heal in days or months without any specific treatment. If this doesn't happen, an operation known as a myringoplasty is often recommended, in which the perforation is closed; nine times out of ten this is successfully achieved. The aim of the operation is to reduce the chance of recurrent infections; sometimes hearing is improved as well.

In a standard myringoplasty, performed under general anesthetic, the surgeon covers the perforation with a graft of temporalis fascia (connective tissue taken from the temporalis muscle just above the ear). The graft, which is held in place on the eardrum by an absorbable sponge

Microsurgery on the ear

A surgeon uses a microscope to perform an operation on an ear. The monitor shows the surgeon's view: He is going in through the ear canal. A common operation is the repair of a perforated eardrum that has not healed naturally. The example shown at right was caused by an attempt to remove wax with a cotton swab; the blood is from a cut in the canal.

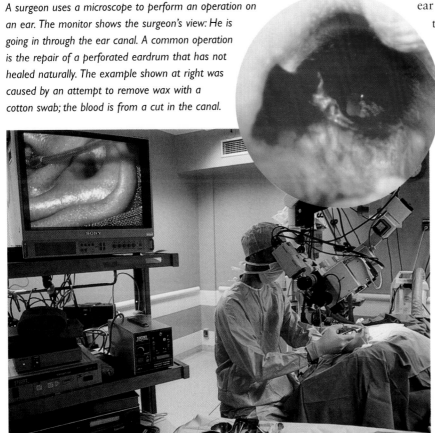

dressing, acts as a scaffold for new blood vessels and skin to grow across. It can take as long as three months for the eardrum to heal fully.

SURGERY ON THE OSSICLES

Hearing loss is sometimes caused by failure of the ossicles —three small bones in the middle ear called the malleus, incus, and stapes—to transmit sound from the eardrum to the inner ear. Failure can result from ossicular erosion following chronic middle ear disease, a fracture of the ossicles, or the ossicular chain having fused together (often caused by otosclerosis). An ossiculoplasty or stapedectomy may be recommended to restore hearing.

Ossiculoplasty

In ossiculoplasty, the surgeon lifts the eardrum to reveal the ossicles and then replaces the damaged ossicle with a refashioned one made on the spot from the old, damaged ossicle, or from bone or cartilage taken from elsewhere in the patient's body, or with a synthetic prosthesis. Once the new ossicle is in position, the eardrum is replaced and then held in place with a dressing in the ear canal. It takes 6–12 weeks for the ear to heal fully, and only then can the improvement in hearing be assessed.

Stapedectomy

A stapedectomy involves removing part of the stapes, the innermost of the three ossicles. The surgeon then drills a tiny hole in the immobile stapes footplate in the remaining part of the stapes and fits a pistonlike prosthesis to replace the missing part. This prosthesis takes over the stapes's function of transmitting sound from the incus (the middle ossicle) to the inner ear. Although the operation is quoted as having a 98 percent success rate, it is not without risk: Damage to the inner ear can cause hearing loss, tinnitus, and dizziness. The risk varies from surgeon to surgeon: It is quite legitimate to inquire about a particular surgeon's success rate for this operation.

MASTOID SURGERY

A mastoidectomy is often performed to remove infected matter from the mastoid (the bony protrusion behind the ear and the air space that connects it to the middle ear) and the cavity of the middle ear itself. A typical condition requiring a mastoidectomy is cholesteatoma, which develops when dead, infected skin cells accumulate in the middle ear and mastoid. The surgeon goes in through an incision behind the ear and drills part of the mastoid bone to expose the diseased area and allow removal of the dead tissue. Often, diseased ossicles must be taken out at the same time; this is likely to cause moderate deafness but is necessary if the operation is to be successful.

If the surgeon is able to leave the ear canal intact and the eardrum in position (in what is known as the "canal-wall-up" technique), the possibility of reconstructing the ossicles at a later date remains open, as long as the ear stays free of disease. Sometimes the surgeon has to resort to the more radical "canal-wall-down" technique, however, in which the canal wall must be drilled away to remove the diseased area, leading to enlargement of the ear canal and repositioning of the eardrum. Whichever technique is used, there is a chance that the condition will return and the ear continue to discharge.

> *In the United States, 12 million people have hearing aids, but only half wear them eight hours per day seven days per week.*

HEARING AIDS

Hearing is a complex phenomenon and simply amplifying the surrounding noise electronically is not sufficient. Each aid has to be tailored to the user's pattern of hearing. Often, an aid must be programmed to amplify high-frequency sounds but not to overamplify low-frequency sounds if what the user hears should not be distorted. A common problem is whistling caused by acoustic feedback resulting from the aid not being correctly fitted in the ear.

Almost all hearing aids now issued are battery-powered and use an analog or digital sound system. They are worn behind or inside the ear. For those people who are either unable to wear a standard hearing aid or cannot gain much benefit from one, a surgically implanted hearing aid is often the answer.

Bone-anchored hearing aids

Some patients have diseases of the middle ear that either make it difficult for them to tolerate an earpiece inside the ear, or that block the process of air conduction on which most hearing aids depend. A bone-conducting aid, which transmits sound through the bone behind the ear, can be the solution in such cases. The bone-conducting aid can be worn on a headband, but more convenient is a bone-anchored aid, which is surgically attached to the bone behind the ear. The surgeon implants a titanium screw into the bone of the patient's skull. Six weeks later, the hearing aid is attached to the screw. Bone-anchored aids, introduced in the U.K. in the 1980s, have proven popular there, but they are not commonly used in the U.S. About 5–10 percent of patients have healing problems where the screw protrudes through the skin.

Standard hearing aids

a Sound is picked up by a battery-powered microphone positioned behind the ear, amplified, and then transmitted down a transparent plastic tube into a mold that fits into the concha of the outer ear. The aid has a volume control that the user adjusts manually.

b A hearing aid worn in the ear is less visible, but it requires more manual dexterity to place the aid in the ear and to operate the controls. The small dial controls the volume of incoming sound. The flap is the lid to the battery case.

c A bone-anchored hearing aid sits just behind the ear; it transmits sound through the bone behind the ear, bypassing the middle ear. The aid is held in position by a small titanium fixing that has been surgically attached to the patient's skull and protrudes through the skin.

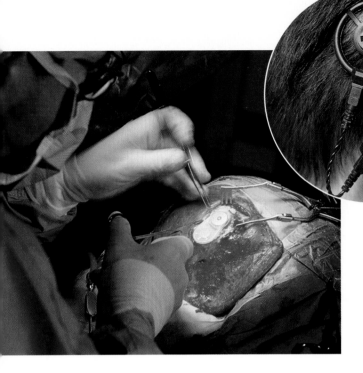

Fitting a cochlear implant
A surgeon places an implant under a flap of skin behind the ear of a patient. Inset: the visible parts of the aid comprise a microphone worn behind the ear that is attached by wires both to a coil held in place above the implant by a magnet and to a speech processor box (not shown here).

with the problem. The process involves cutting through the skin behind the ear to reach the cartilage that forms the shape of the ear. Shape is restored by cutting or scoring the cartilage or bending it to create an antihelical fold and then holding that position with permanent stitches through the cartilage. A head bandage must be left in place for a week to maintain the new shape and prevent excessive bruising.

OCCASIONAL COMPLICATIONS

Although complications after ear surgery are rare, the inner ear and facial nerve are both vulnerable to accidental damage. Surgeons, aware of this, do their best to preserve them. The risks, however, must be considered in context—the diseases for which surgery is performed (such as cholesteatoma and chronic infection) can themselves damage the facial nerve or inner ear or spread infection to the cranial cavity if they go untreated.

Cochlear implants

These devices, in use since the 1970s, provide sound awareness for someone who is profoundly deaf and therefore beyond the reach of a more traditional hearing aid. A microphone worn behind the ear receives the sound; the signal is then processed in a speech processor box worn on a belt or behind the ear, from where it is transmitted to components internally implanted behind the ear; and an electrical signal then travels from the implant to the cochlea via an electrode cable that has been inserted directly into the cochlea of the inner ear.

About half of all cochlear implantees gain a good degree of speech discrimination; some can even use the telephone. However, it can take years of training and practice to get the maximum benefit from the implant.

Totally implantable middle ear hearing aids

Available only since the early 2000s, these aids are fitted into the middle ear, where they are attached to the incus (the middle ossicle). The surgeon gains access through the mastoid bone. Hearing results are good when compared to a patient's previous aids, but the implant is costly and requires a complex operation with attendant risks.

SURGERY FOR PROMINENT EARS

A common congenital deformity of the ear is a failure of development of the antihelical fold (the bend in the wing of the outer ear that molds an ear so it follows the shape of the head). As a result, the ears appear very prominent. In such cases, an operation called a otoplasty can deal

ON THE CUTTING EDGE

Digital hearing aids

Digital hearing aids can be worn in or behind the ear. They work by taking a sound signal and converting it into data that are manipulated by a computer in the aid. In this way, sound can be processed precisely and the hearing aid adjusted to suit each user. In general, digital aids perform better than analog aids. But users of analog aids, convinced that a digital aid is the answer to problems with hearing speech against a noisy background, are often not getting the best out of their analog hearing aids. With time and practice, many users of analog aids are able to automatically "screen out" more obtrusive background noises than they could to begin with.

Removing nasal polyps

The latest and most complete way of removing nasal polyps is by means of endoscopic sinus surgery, in which cutting edge surgical instruments enable a surgeon to remove polyps entirely with minimal trauma to the nose itself.

Nasal polyps tend to occur in patients with rhinitis. Rare in children, they are more common in men than women. They are normally benign, resulting only in some loss of smell or blocked breathing. When they are removed, it is generally because they form an obstruction within the nose. Rarely, a benign or malignant sinus tumor can create polyps, usually on one side of the nose.

Nasal polyps are treated either with steroid medications or with surgery and often with a combination of both. The surgeon usually requests a CT scan of the sinuses to determine the extent of the disease and to help plan any operations.

The simplest surgical procedure is an intranasal polypectomy—removal of polyps from the nasal passages under local or general anesthetic. The operation improves breathing and, to a variable degree, the patient's sense of smell, but there is a possibility that the polyps will return.

Endoscopic sinus surgery

More extensive surgery removes the polyps not just from the nose but also from the sinuses where they originate, thus decreasing the chances of recurrence. Endoscopic sinus surgery (ESS) enables the surgeon to follow the disease into the sinuses and remove it entirely.

Endoscopic sinus surgery has largely replaced the more traditional sinus operations, in which surgical cuts were made on the face or under the upper lip. Disadvantages of traditional "open" sinus surgery include external scarring, greater bruising and discomfort, and more bleeding. However, traditional "open" surgery is still regarded as the most efficient option in some circumstances, such as when a tumor must be removed from the sinuses.

The surgical procedure

1 The nasal polyp that is to be cut out is clearly visible and totally blocking the patient's nostril. It originates in the maxillary sinus, and will be removed using minimally invasive techniques known as endoscopic sinus surgery (ESS). As soon as the patient has been anesthetized, the nasal lining is prepared for surgery with medications that decongest the mucous membrane. This helps improve visibility and reduce bleeding.

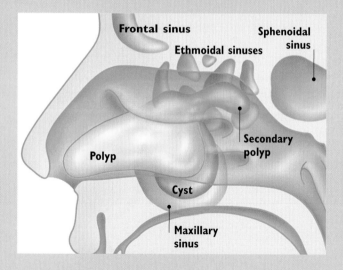

Frontal sinus

Sphenoidal sinus

Ethmoidal sinuses

Secondary polyp

Polyp

Cyst

Maxillary sinus

Polyps within the nose and sinuses

Nasal polyps are round, smooth, soft, swollen, semi-translucent structures that appear singly or in a cluster that can resemble a small bunch of grapes. Polyps originate in the swollen or prolapsed lining of one of the paranasal sinuses, to which they are attached by a stalk. They extend into the nasal cavity and, often, down one or both nostrils. They most commonly develop in the ethmoidal sinuses, a collection of air-filled spaces within the ethmoid bone (between the nose and the floor of the cavity containing the brain). Sometimes a polyp is attached to a cyst positioned at the opening of one of the maxillary sinuses.

3

2

4

5

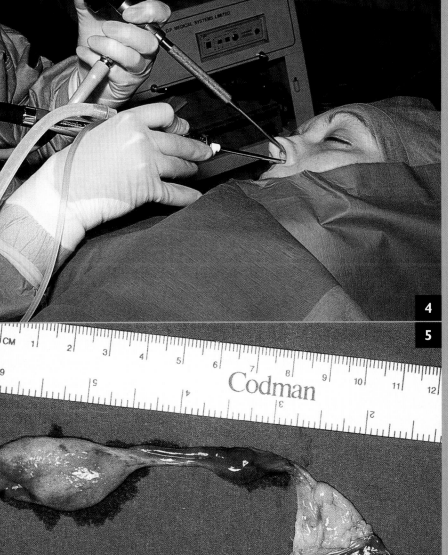

2 By inserting a rigid 0.16-inch endoscope into the nostril in which the polyp is growing, the surgeon can clearly visualize the inside of the nose. The tip of the endoscope is fitted with a fiberoptic light that illuminates the operation site and a high-resolution camera that transmits an image of the site to a large viewing monitor. Throughout the operation, the surgeon is able to see the site and monitor the progress of the operation on the screen.

3 A secondary polyp in the back of the nose, with surrounding infection, is identified and displayed on the monitor.

4 Working parallel to the endoscope (held in her left hand), the surgeon can introduce a variety of instruments into the same nostril. Specialized angled instruments allow access to all the nasal sinuses, but here a powered debrider is being used to cut and aspirate away targeted tissue while leaving the surrounding mucous membrane untouched. The suction tubing keeps the operation site clear.

5 The main body of the polyp, now removed, is a surprising 1.5 inches long. It is attached to a large cyst that was removed from the left maxillary sinus.

Nose and sinus surgery

A variety of conditions affecting the nose and sinuses, from congenital defects to severe cases of rhinitis, require surgery. Microscopes and endoscopes have revolutionized surgical procedures in these areas, making them safer and more effective than ever before.

TREATING RHINITIS

Most cases of rhinitis—inflammation of the lining of the nose—are treated with medication (see page 118). Some cases, however, can require surgical intervention such as with rhinitis caused by chronic swelling of the turbinates (ridges covered with mucous membrane) within the nasal cavity. A local anesthetic is applied and a laser or electrocautery is used to reduce the swelling.

CORRECTING A DEVIATED SEPTUM

The nasal septum is the cartilage and bone partition that separates the nostrils. A deviated—or twisted—septum reduces airflow through the nasal passages; it generally affects one side more than the other. A deviated septum may be congenital or result from an injury such as a blow to the nose. Surgery under general anesthetic should solve the problem. There are two main types of operation.

- Submucous resection of the nasal septum Deviated bone and cartilage is removed from under the lining of the septum, and then the lining is replaced.
- Septoplasty In this procedure, a minimal amount of the distorted cartilage and bone is removed and the remaining parts are realigned in the center.

Nasal–septal perforation

There should be no internal communication between the two sides of the nose. Occasionally, a connection between the two sides—a nasal–septal perforation—occurs, but this rarely causes problems. If it does, graft techniques are used to close it.

Aesthetic nasal surgery

Rhinoplasty is the most common aesthetic surgical procedure in the United States. Rhinoplasty reshapes or rebalances the nose and can have a dramatic impact on a person's appearance and self-esteem. The majority of requests are for nasal reduction. Most aesthetic surgery is performed internally via the nostrils, so there is no visible scarring.

Choosing to have nose surgery is a personal decision and not one to make lightly. A reputable surgeon will advise you on what can be achieved in each individual

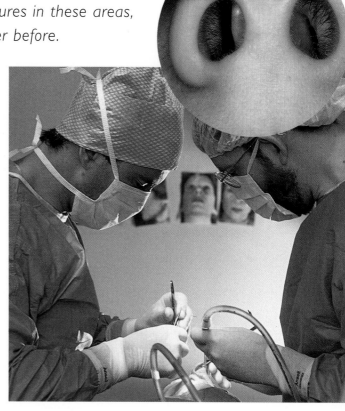

Plastic surgery on the nose
Rhinoplasty—surgery to alter the shape or internal structure of the nose—is performed either to correct a problem that affects the nose's ability to function properly, such as a twisted septum (shown top, between the two nostrils), or for purely aesthetic reasons (above).

case. Anyone performing such surgery should specialize in facial plastic surgery and be a member of the American Academy of Facial Plastic and Reconstructive Surgery.

SURGERY FOR RECURRENT SINUSITIS

In some patients prone to recurrent sinus infections, the connecting passages between the nose and sinuses are too narrow. To enlarge these openings and improve drainage through the natural pathways into the nose, the technique known as functional endoscopic sinus surgery (FESS) is employed. By using an endoscope to view the sinus openings on a monitor, a surgeon is able to enlarge the sinus openings, using a cutting tool introduced into the nasal cavity via a nostril. FESS leaves no external scars and can be performed under local or general anesthetic.

Throat surgery

The throat forms a passageway through which you breathe, eat, and speak. Surgery on this vital part of the body is a common procedure for an otolaryngologist, with operations ranging from routine tonsillectomies to life-saving tracheostomies.

REMOVING THE TONSILS

The tonsils are at the back of the throat, positioned opposite each other, and attached to the side walls; their surgical removal is known as a tonsillectomy. They are made of the lymphoid tissue that forms part of the body's defense against infection. But because there is sufficient lymphoid tissue elsewhere in the upper respiratory tract to substitute for what has been removed, patients usually develop fewer throat infections after a tonsillectomy rather than more, as might logically be expected. This is because a major focus of infection has been removed.

When is a tonsillectomy recommended?

- **Acute tonsillitis** Tonsils can become subject to a series of attacks of acute tonsillitis caused by repeated infection. Symptoms include a prolonged, severe sore throat with swollen, inflamed tonsils, plus difficulty in swallowing, fever, and a general feeling of being ill. A tonsillectomy—suggested in severe cases—won't prevent another sore throat but will bring an end to these acute attacks.

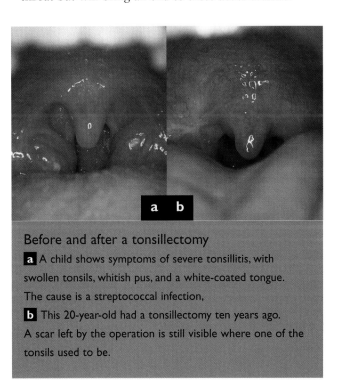

Before and after a tonsillectomy

a A child shows symptoms of severe tonsillitis, with swollen tonsils, whitish pus, and a white-coated tongue. The cause is a streptococcal infection.

b This 20-year-old had a tonsillectomy ten years ago. A scar left by the operation is still visible where one of the tonsils used to be.

- **Enlarged tonsils** Children with enlarged tonsils can find it difficult to sleep properly because the tonsils obstruct their breathing. To improve the breathing, a surgeon may recommend removal of the tonsils, and often the adenoids as well, if they are also enlarged.
- **Draining a quinsy** A peritonsillar abscess, also known as a quinsy, develops when pus—produced as part of the body's reaction to an infection—collects between a tonsil and the muscles of the throat. It may be possible to drain the abscess using a needle or by means of a cut made under local anesthetic. In some cases the surgeon will recommend a tonsillectomy, to be performed either at the time of draining the abscess or after it has settled.
- **Removal of a tumor** Very occasionally, a single enlarged tonsil is a sign of a tumor. This may be a lymphoma (a tumor originating in lymphatic tissue) or a squamous carcinoma (a tumor originating in the lining of the throat and most commonly occurring in smokers).

The operation and afterward

A tonsillectomy is performed under general anesthetic. With the mouth held open by a retractor, the tonsils are carefully dissected and removed. Bleeding is stopped with electrocautery or by surgical ties. The patient generally leaves the hospital the day of or the day after the operation with a sore throat that usually lasts about 7 to 10 days.

Stuck in the throat
This side view X-ray shows a safety pin that was accidentally swallowed. Sharp foreign bodies form a particular danger when lodged in the esophagus, because they can perforate the esophageal walls.

REMOVING THE ADENOIDS

The adenoids form another collection of lymphoid tissue, similar to that in the tonsils. They are found in the region behind the nose called the nasopharynx. They generally shrink in size during adolescence, so children will often outgrow any adenoidal problems. However, some conditions need to be dealt with sooner rather than later —in these cases the solution is often an adenoidectomy.

When is an adenoidectomy recommended?

- Enlarged adenoids The passage of air through the eustachian tube, which connects the ear to the throat, can be obstructed by enlarged adenoids. When this regularly disrupts a child's sleep, surgery may be the answer.
- Middle ear infections There is increasing evidence that removing the adenoids may reduce the duration of middle ear infections. The operation is often combined with the insertion of ear tubes.
- Infected adenoids Until recently, children with rhinitis coupled with a general feeling of being unwell were likely to be diagnosed as having chronically infected adenoids; the cure was to have the adenoids cut out. Nowadays, these symptoms are often diagnosed as an allergic response that is more effectively treated by other means. A deep-seated infection of the adenoids is still sometimes treated by their removal, however.

The operation

An adenoidectomy is performed under general anesthetic and usually takes less than 15 minutes. Operating through the mouth with the aid of a mirror, the surgeon shaves away layers of adenoidal tissue. Electrocautery keeps bleeding to a minimum. The tonsils are often removed at the same time, but if the adenoids alone are excised, the patient's throat is much less sore afterward.

FOREIGN BODIES IN THE THROAT

All sorts of objects can lodge in the throat—small bones, nuts, and coins are common examples. If these don't clear by themselves, they have to be removed surgically. The procedure depends on what the object is and where it is stuck. As well as being swallowed, foreign bodies can be inhaled and lodge in the larynx (voice box), trachea (windpipe), or bronchi (airways from the trachea to the lungs). A small bone lodged in a tonsil is easily removed with forceps after a spray of local anesthetic. Removing an object farther down the throat often requires a general anesthetic. After locating the object by means of an X-ray or a flexible endoscope passed down the throat, the surgeon retrieves it with grasping forceps attached to an endoscope or rigid bronchoscope.

REMOVING SINGER'S NODULES AND POLYPS

Nodules—almost always benign—appear on the vocal cords in pairs, one on each cord. These tiny, hardened, gray–white lumps develop on the cords of people—often singers or teachers (hence, their name)—who habitually overuse their voices and so strain their vocal cords. It is generally hoarseness that sends them to the doctor. Treatment involves resting the voice, speech therapy, and avoiding irritants such as cigarette smoke. With this treatment, the nodules will shrink and hopefully disappear. If the nodules fail to shrink sufficiently or are very large to begin with, they are removed surgically. Viewing a magnified image of the vocal cords, the surgeon uses a laryngoscope with a carbon dioxide laser or scalpel to remove the nodes.

One or more polyps on the cords appear as smooth, rounded swellings. Like nodules, they are generally benign. The symptoms, causes, and initial treatment are usually the same as for nodules. However, most polyps end up having to be removed surgically (following procedures similar to those used when removing nodules). Polyps and nodules can return if the patient does not modify poor voice habits and strains the voice again.

TRACHEOSTOMY

Tracheostomy is a procedure that creates an opening in the neck into which a tube is inserted that enters the trachea below the larynx and vocal cords. The aim is to maintain the passage of air to the lungs. The patient breathes in and out through the open tracheostomy tube. A tracheostomy tube may be inserted because

- the airway is obstructed higher up;
- the patient must use an artificial ventilator for help with breathing all or part of the time;
- the patient has problems with fluids entering the airway from the throat; or
- the airway opening has to be rerouted as part of a major operation involving the head and neck.

The tracheostomy tube

1 Having made an incision in the skin of the patient's neck, the surgeon cuts through to the trachea (windpipe) to form an opening known as a stoma, and then inserts a short length of tube to maintain the opening.

2 Once the tracheostomy tube is in place it can be attached to a ventilator that administers the general anesthetic during an operation.

3 When the tracheostomy tube is open, as it is here, air enters and leaves the lungs via the tube. When the tube is shut, air enters and leaves the lungs via the nose or mouth. To maintain the stoma, the tube must be kept in place. To reverse the tracheostomy, the tube is simply removed and the opening begins to close over within a few days.

Can you speak after a tracheostomy?

Breathing through a tracheostomy tube means that air is diverted before it reaches the vocal cords. Because a stream of air is needed for the vocal cords to work, a patient with an open tracheostomy tube can't use his or her vocal cords to produce the sounds needed for speech. However, most patients who undergo a tracheostomy can manage to speak satisfactorily. Some patients have a tube that is covered most of the time; for them, speech is not a problem. Others can cover the opening whenever they want to speak. For others, the solution depends on the nature of the problem. For example, someone with a tracheostomy because the airway is only partially obstructed may be able to breathe with the help of a smaller-than-normal tube, so that with each exhalation some air exits via the tube and some passes through the vocal cords.

ASK THE EXPERT

When the airway is obstructed

The airway can become obstructed by a foreign body or as a result of injury, an infection, or a disease such as cancer. The airway can only be completely blocked for a few minutes before brain damage starts to take place, so a tracheostomy may need to be carried out as an emergency bypass of the blockage. More often, however, there is a gradual onset to the airway obstruction, allowing time to plan a tracheostomy in advance.

When the patient is dependent on a ventilator

A tracheostomy is often performed on patients who cannot breathe naturally and require artificial ventilation (pumping of air into the lungs by a machine) either all or part of the time. If the patient has not had a tracheostomy, a ventilation tube is passed down the larynx and into the upper trachea via the mouth or nose. This is so uncomfortable that the patient usually has to be sedated while artificial ventilation takes place.

Attaching the ventilation tube to a tracheostomy tube instead brings a number of benefits: The patient can breathe without sedation; it becomes easier to wean the patient from a ventilator; and the airway is no longer in danger of becoming scarred or permanently narrowed by prolonged use of the ventilation tube.

Removing head and neck tumors

The surgery performed on head and neck tumors (principally cancers of the throat, mouth, or tongue) is often life-saving. Specialists are on hand every step of the way to help patients through the operation and support them on their journey back to health.

LOCATION AND TREATMENT

Each year, about 40,000 patients in the United States develop cancer of the head and neck. Most cases are of a type known as squamous cell carcinoma, principally caused by smoking. Cancers can occur anywhere in the lining of the mouth, throat, or larynx (voice box), and treatment depends on the location, size, and spread of the tumor. In general, squamous cell carcinomas first spread from the primary site to the lymph glands in the neck; in approximately 5 in 100 cases, they spread to more distant regions of the body, such as the lungs, liver, or bones. The recommended treatment is usually surgery, radiation, or a combination of both. In certain instances, chemotherapy may also be recommended.

> *Head and neck cancers account for 3 percent of all cancers; 85 percent of head and neck cancers can be linked to tobacco use.*

SURGERY ON THE VOCAL CORDS

One of the most common lesions is a tumor of the vocal cords within the larynx. These are usually spotted early, because even a very small growth will make the patient's voice sound hoarse. Tumors may need removal using microsurgical techniques, often performed with a laser. A relatively good quality of voice is usually regained following surgery. An alternative treatment for small vocal cord tumors is radiation.

LARYNGECTOMY

Larger tumors of the larynx, or those that recur after radiation, require more extensive surgery. This may mean the partial or total removal of the larynx—an operation referred to as a laryngectomy. A partial laryngectomy may be performed by means of an endoscopic laser technique or via an incision in the neck. If the latter course is taken, a temporary tracheostomy is often necessary. If the entire larynx has to be cut out,

the tracheostomy is permanent. Following a total laryngectomy, therefore, the patient is unable to speak and must breathe through the opening in the neck created by the tracheostomy (see page 129).

Regaining speech after a laryngectomy

The vast majority of patients regain some form of speech following a laryngectomy, and there are several ways they can achieve this with the help of regular practice under the supervision of a specially trained speech therapist.

• A speech valve This usually produces the best results as far as voice quality is concerned. The valve is implanted at the back of the windpipe. A patient who wants to speak places a finger over the open tracheostomy tube and breathes out; air

A speech therapist at work
A patient who has undergone a tracheostomy as part of a laryngectomy, and so has lost her vocal cords, learns to talk again using esophageal speech, with the help of a speech therapist.

that would normally exit via the tube passes into the throat and through the valve, which resonates in a similar way to the vocal cords.

- **Esophageal speech** The basic idea is to swallow air and then regurgitate it to produce speech; in fact, esophageal speech resembles an energetic form of burping. Quite intelligible speech can be produced by this method, but sentences often have to be kept short.
- **An electrolarynx** This is an electrical source of vibration. Holding the battery-operated device against the neck, the patient speaks in a normal manner and the device translates this into an electronic monotone voice. The speech can be understood but has a metallic, tinny quality that some patients don't feel comfortable with.

SURGERY ON THE TONGUE AND PHARYNX

Tumors of the tongue and pharynx (the muscular tube leading from the back of the nose and mouth to the top of the esophagus) are often removed along with part or all of the surrounding area. This can have an effect on the patient's ability to swallow. Small operations may produce a temporary problem; more extensive procedures can necessitate careful reconstruction of the swallowing passage, using muscles from the chest wall or pieces of the intestine or stomach and skin from the arm or leg. Once healed, these can work as well as the original passage structure.

Learning to swallow again

Throughout the healing process, the patient is fed through a tube, which is usually passed up the nose or directly into the stomach through the abdomen. While in the hospital, patients are shown how to use the feeding tube and associated equipment, so that they can manage them at home. Regular sessions with a speech therapist—also an expert on swallowing—help the patient to recover the ability to swallow. Following a swallowing assessment, which may take the form of a video X-ray examination or an endoscope-guided examination (see page 111) of the swallowing mechanism, the therapist will advise on maneuvers and exercises that will help a patient regain the ability to swallow and do without the feeding tube.

Cancer in the lymph glands
In this colored single-photon CT scan of a head, lymph glands invaded by cells that are cancerous show up yellow and red.

SURGERY FOR CANCEROUS LYMPH NODES

Foreign swellings that have spread to the lymph glands of the neck can be treated by surgical removal or radiation. The choice of treatment is based on a number of factors. The site and size, as well as the type of treatment given for the initial tumor, are important. For example, larger lumps in the neck are often treated surgically. The tumor pathology report will influence the decision, as will the number of neck glands affected, and whether the tumor has spread outside the lymph glands.

Neck dissection

An operation in which the lymph glands are removed from one side of the neck is known as a neck dissection. The extent of the neck dissection depends on the location and size of the primary tumor. There are about 200 lymph glands in the neck; in a typical neck dissection, between 30 and 50 glands might be removed.

The operation is performed through an incision in the neck. Although great care is taken not to damage any nerves, blood vessels, or muscles, this can be unavoidable. For instance, if the major nerve to the shoulder (called the spinal accessory nerve) is affected by the disease, it may have to be cut. This causes some stiffness in the shoulders and weakness in the muscles used to shrug the shoulder, and is followed with physical therapy. In some cases the large muscle of the neck, the sternocleidomastoid, may be removed. This generally changes the contour of the neck, leaving a hollowed-out profile on one side.

A LUMP IN THE THYROID GLAND

A lump in the neck is sometimes, in fact, a lump in the thyroid gland. This is an endocrine gland that manufactures and secretes hormones into the bloodstream. It consists of two lobes on either side of the Adam's apple at the top of the trachea connected by a narrow band of thyroid tissue known as the isthmus.

The lump or lumps may be cancerous or benign. To find out, the doctor will begin by ordering a fine-needle aspiration cytology (FNAC) test (see page 112), plus an ultrasound scan. When the diagnosis is cancer of the thyroid, a surgeon will generally remove part or all of the thyroid gland; the function of the gland is replaced by the patient taking thyroid hormone—generally in pill form—every day for the rest of his or her life. Follow-up treatment to eliminate remaining cancer cells depends on the type and extent of the cancer, but may include doses of radioactive iodine or external beam radiation. Radioactive iodine is either swallowed or injected into a vein in the arm; only thyroid cells—both cancerous and healthy—will absorb the iodine and so inevitably receive a high dose of radiation as well.

A benign lump is also often removed, at least partially, because of the risk of it compressing any of the crucial structures in the neck, especially the trachea.

A lump may be a symptom of the thyroid gland being overactive and producing too much thyroid hormone. Removing part of the thyroid was once the most common treatment, but this has been largely replaced by the use of radioactive iodine and various drugs to bring the amount of hormones produced down to a normal level.

THE COMBINED HEAD AND NECK CLINIC

At some point, a patient with a head or neck tumor will probably be referred to a special combined clinic for head and neck complaints. Here the patient will see a variety of specialists including surgeons, oncologists (specialists in the treatment of tumors), specialist nurses, speech therapists, radiologists, dietitians, and physical therapists. Each specialist contributes to designing a total treatment program for the patient, taking into account the nature, size, and site of the tumor.

- Clinical nurse specialists Not only can these nurses help with pain control, dressings, and so forth, but they are a key point of contact for a patient if new problems arise. They may well have received training as specialists in cancer treatment and care.
- Physical therapists Shoulder and neck pain and stiffness are common following head and neck surgery and physical therapy can often help.
- Dietitians Maintaining a healthy diet and body weight is difficult when the ability to swallow is limited—perhaps so limited that the patient can only consume liquids. The dietitian works out the best diet for each patient

and in what form it is best taken. Patients with feeding tubes need guidance on how often and for how long they must feed via the tube to get the nutrients they need.

EXTERNAL BEAM RADIATION

External beam radiation is a key treatment for tumors of the head and neck. This involves controlled doses of ionizing radiation that slow or destroy the development of abnormal cells in diseased tissue. It is given either on its own, before or after surgery, and is usually carried out over six weeks, with the patient visiting the clinic most weekdays.

Information gained from scans and examinations of the tumor with an endoscope will have determined which regions to irradiate. During the patient's first visit, treatments are discussed and a mold is made of the patient's head and neck. At each subsequent visit, the patient's head is fixed in position by a clear plastic mask and a very precise dose of radiation is delivered to the area that requires treatment.

To reduce side effects, the amount of radiation delivered to the area surrounding the tumor is kept to an absolute minimum. Despite this, some patients who undergo head and neck radiation complain of a permanently dry mouth and throat, a troublesome feeling that can last for months or even years. This is caused by radiation disturbing the salivary glands that keep the mouth and throat moist. An artificial salivary product will ease this side effect, as will frequent sips of water.

A patient receives radiation
A custom-made plastic mask is used during every dose of radiation to ensure that the patient's head is always in exactly the same position, so that precisely the same spot is exposed to the radiation every time.

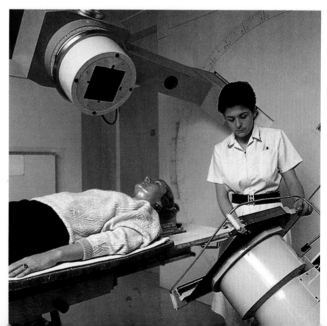

A TO Z

OF DISEASES AND DISORDERS

This section gives information on the main illnesses and medical conditions that can affect the ears, nose, and throat.

This index is arranged alphabetically and each entry is structured in a similar way:

What are the causes?

What are the symptoms?

How is it diagnosed?

What are the treatment options?

What is the outlook?

ACOUSTIC NEUROMA

A benign tumor on the nerve that carries balance and hearing from the inner ear to the brain.

An acoustic neuroma (also known as a vestibular schwannoma) is a growth on part of the nerve that is involved in balance and hearing. The growth is benign—it is not a cancer—but because of its proximity to the brain, it can have serious effects if it grows to be very large.

What are the symptoms?

The most common symptom is a gradual loss of hearing in one ear. Other less common symptoms include
- tinnitus;
- balance problems; and
- facial pain, numbness, or tingling.

Very large tumors may cause headaches, double vision, facial paralysis, and (rarely) drowsiness.

How is it diagnosed?

A hearing test is often the first investigation. This will show up any hearing loss in the affected ear. An MRI scan of the head (p. 115) is then the best investigation to detect an acoustic neuroma. For patients who are unable to undergo MRI scanning, a CT scan may be appropriate, with or without tests of auditory function called brainstem response audiometry.

Severe claustrophobia or a surgical implant such as a pacemaker may make a patient unsuitable for MRI scanning.

What are the treatment options?

Each case is assessed on its own merits, taking into consideration factors such as the size and position of the tumor, the age and general health of the patient, and the patient's preferences for treatment.

Surgery aims for total removal of the tumor with as little damage to surrounding brain tissue and nerves as possible. Recovery from surgery can take up to three months and some degree of hearing loss or facial nerve paralysis is not uncommon. However, once removed totally, the tumor is unlikely to return.

Stereotactic radiosurgery, or the gamma knife, is a form of radiation in which the beams are focused specifically on the small area of tumor. In this way, radiation to surrounding tissues is minimized. This is suitable only for smaller tumors, and in some cases the tumor may not disappear completely but may shrink or its growth may be stopped.

If the tumor grows very slowly, it may be worth monitoring the tumor with regular scans before treatment is considered, because the risks of treatment can be greater than the problems the tumor is causing.

What is the outlook?

Acoustic neuromas tend to be slow-growing tumors, so decisions about treatment do not have to be rushed. Intensive rehabilitation after surgery will get most people back to a full and active life.

BAROTRAUMA

The effect that changes in atmospheric pressure have on the ear.

Changes in air pressure, such as those encountered flying or scuba diving, can cause ear pain and hearing problems.

What is the cause?

Barotrauma is caused by a failure to equalize the pressure of the middle ear with the pressure of the external surroundings caused by poor eustachian tube function. The eustachian tube, which runs from the back of the nose to the middle ear, normally allows air into and out of the ear to keep the pressure equal to atmospheric pressure. This produces the popping sensation we normally feel in the ears with pressure changes.

What are the symptoms?

As atmospheric pressure changes, for example on descent in an airplane, the ear becomes painful and fails to pop to clear. Hearing is usually muffled. These symptoms often resolve spontaneously within hours or days, but they may persist, particularly if the barotrauma has caused fluid to collect in the middle ear (an effusion).

How is it diagnosed?

Examination of the ear using an otoscope may reveal fluid or blood behind the eardrum. This may be confirmed by a hearing test and a test to measure the movement of the eardrum and middle ear pressure, known as tympanometry (p. 108).

What are the treatment options?

Prevention can be important for people who are known to have suffered problems in the past. People should avoid flying if they have a severe cold or upper respiratory tract infection. Sucking on hard candy or sipping a drink during takeoff and descent can help, as can nasal decongestants taken before the journey.

Divers should be trained to equalize middle ear pressure during a dive and should avoid diving if they cannot do so. A myringotomy—making a small hole in the eardrum—to drain any residual fluid can treat persistent deafness. An ear tube (p. 120) can be inserted if necessary, for example in frequent flyers with recurrent problems.

BROKEN NOSE
A fracture of the nasal bones.

This is a common result of a blow to the nose, which may result from assault, car accident, or sports injury.

What are the symptoms?
Once the bruising and swelling caused by the injury disappear, there may be no obvious sign of a fracture. The nose may remain tender to touch for a few weeks, and there may be a change in the shape of the nose.

How is it diagnosed?
Most fractures are diagnosed by talking to the patient and physically examining the nose. X-rays are required only if other injuries of the bones of the face are suspected or if evidence of the fracture is required for legal purposes, if criminal proceedings may occur, for example.

What are the treatment options?
If there is no deformity of the nose after the swelling has gone down, usually about one week after receiving the injury, no treatment is necessary. If there is an obvious change in the shape of the nose, manipulation of the bones under general anesthetic may be necessary. This is usually performed within two weeks of the injury before the bones have fully set. If the shape cannot be corrected by simple manipulation, cosmetic surgery, or rhinoplasty, may be required.

CANCER OF THE LARYNX
Cancer affecting the area of the throat around and including the voice box.

In the West, this is the most common cancer affecting the head and neck; there are about 12,000 cases each year in the U.S.

What is the cause?
Certain factors, smoking and heavy alcohol consumption in particular, are known to trigger the changes in cells that lead to cancer.

What are the symptoms?
A hoarse voice that does not get better is the most common and often the only symptom. Other symptoms include difficulty swallowing and breathing, pain in the throat or ear, and sometimes a lump in the neck.

How is it diagnosed?
The larynx can be examined in the ENT office either using a mirror or a flexible endoscope. If a suspicious area is seen, a biopsy needs to be performed; this is done under a general anesthetic. Scans of the throat and neck, along with the biopsy findings, will help determine the most suitable treatment.

What are the treatment options?
Treatment depends upon the exact site and size of the tumor, on whether there is any spread to the neck glands, and on the health and preferences of the patient.

Radiation is appropriate for some smaller tumors. On average, a course of treatment lasts six weeks. It is also sometimes given after surgical treatment if it is felt there is a risk that the tumor may recur.

Surgery can vary from localized treatment, such as laser surgery for small tumors, to more extensive operations, such as laryngectomy, for larger tumors. Laryngectomy involves removing the voice box and part of the windpipe, leaving a small hole or stoma in the neck for breathing.

If the tumor is very large, part of the top of the esophagus may also need to be removed and tissue is then taken from other parts of the body to repair this. Rehabilitation after such surgery involves relearning swallowing and speech. Despite the surgical removal of the voice box, many patients achieve an excellent "voice" with the help of a speech therapist.

If the disease has spread to the neck, surgery may be required to remove the lymph nodes; this is usually performed at the same time.

What is the outlook?
Five-year survival for this cancer is 50–60 percent. The outlook for individual patients depends on the extent of the tumor at the time of diagnosis. At initial diagnosis, 95 percent of patients are treatable, although not all are

Medicine, surgery, radiation, and chemotherapy all control symptoms and ease cancer pain.

curable. Patients who have had treatment are followed up closely at regular intervals to detect any sign of the return of the cancer so that further treatment can be planned quickly if it should become necessary.

CANCER OF THE NASOPHARYNX
A tumor of the area at the back of the nose.

The nasopharynx is the area at the back of the nose above the palate. Although cancer can occur in people of any race, in this area it is most common among people of Chinese ethnicity. There may be a genetic element to the disease, but modifiable risk factors include avoiding salted fish (an Asian staple from infancy) and fermented foods.

What are the symptoms?
Many patients have no symptoms until the tumor is very large. Many complain of nasal blockage, nosebleeds, or a lump in the neck. The tumor may block the eustachian tube, leading to a buildup of fluid and deafness.

How is it diagnosed?
The nasopharynx can be examined in the ENT office using a mirror or an endoscope. If there is any suspicion that there is a tumor present, a biopsy is performed under general anesthetic, usually in the operating room. Scans can be useful in planning treatment.

What are the treatment options?
Radiation with chemotherapy is the treatment of choice. Surgery is occasionally necessary to remove the neck glands if the disease has spread to them.

What is the outlook?
Depending on the extent of the disease when a patient is first diagnosed, five-year survival can be up to 90 percent.

DEVIATED NASAL SEPTUM
A bent or misshapen septum—the partition in the nose that divides it into left and right cavities.

What is the cause?
The septum may become bent following an accident or during growth of the nose in childhood.

What are the symptoms?
The nose will feel blocked on the narrower side, and the deviation may sometimes cause external twisting of the shape of the nose.

What is the treatment?
If treatment is required to relieve the blockage, surgery is indicated. The operation is called a septoplasty or sub-mucous resection of the septum. The septum is made of cartilage and bone, and this can be straightened from inside the nose by removing some of the tissue and repositioning the rest. This is commonly performed under a general anesthetic.

What is the outlook?
Recovery from surgery is usually quick. For the first week to ten days, there is a little discomfort in the nose, described by most people as feeling like a blockage or pressure. There is a small chance of infection in the nose for a week after surgery—after all, the nose is not the cleanest of areas—which can lead to bleeding, known as secondary hemorrhage. This does not seem to be prevented by giving prophylactic antibiotics, but an infection should respond well to a course of treatment.

Although surgery to correct a deviated septum requires a general anesthetic, patients can usually go home the same day.

The nose should be healed, and the patient should be able to resume normal activities within two weeks of surgery.

EPIGLOTTITIS
Inflammation of the epiglottis due to infection.

The epiglottis is a leaf-shaped structure in the throat that helps close the airway during swallowing to prevent food and drink going down the "wrong way" into the lungs. Inflammation of this structure is called epiglottitis.

What is the cause?
Infection is caused by bacteria and occurs most commonly in children between 2 and 6 years old, but it can occur in adults. The pattern of incidence is changing since the introduction of the Hib vaccine.

What are the symptoms?
The infection may occur at any time of year but is more common in the winter. The first symptom is usually a sore throat. The epiglottis becomes swollen and the pain

Hib vaccination has virtually eradicated epiglottitis

TALKING POINT

The Hib vaccine was introduced in the United States in 1985 to protect against the *Haemophilus influenzae* bacterium, a primary cause of both epiglottitis and meningitis. Epiglottitis used to be considered a children's disease because it generally affected children aged 3 to 7 years. However, because of the vaccination, it now affects adults more often. The case rate is 1 in 100,000 with a mortality rate of 7 percent for adults. For children, there is only 0.63 case per 100,000 with a mortality rate of less than 1 percent.

becomes more severe so that even swallowing saliva is difficult and the patient drools. The voice becomes muffled, and as swelling increases, breathing becomes difficult and noisy. There is usually a fever.

What are the treatment options?

Medical advice should be sought early, because severe breathing difficulties can occur rapidly. Treatment requires admission to the hospital for intravenous antibiotics and fluids. If breathing difficulties are severe, a tube may need to be inserted through the mouth to help (intubation with an endotracheal tube), or tracheostomy (an incision into the upper air passage) may need to be performed.

What is the outlook?

The infection usually responds rapidly to treatment, and within 48 hours most patients are making a good recovery. There are rarely any long-term consequences following epiglottitis.

EPISTAXIS

A complaint better known as a nosebleed.

What are the causes?

There is no obvious cause for about 85 percent of nosebleeds, which are due to spontaneous rupture of a small blood vessel inside the nose. The remaining 15 percent have a variety of causes, such as trauma to the nose (including picking!), infection, tumors, blood disorders, allergies, and some medicines.

What are the treatment options?

First aid measures can be tried when a nosebleed starts (p. 51). When the blood vessel responsible can be seen at the front of the nose, cauterization may be necessary for nosebleeds that do not stop. This is usually performed under a local anesthetic to the inside of the nose and can be a little uncomfortable. A chemical stick or hot wire is used to seal the burst blood vessel.

If these remedies fail to stop the bleeding, the nose may need to be packed. This is a method of applying pressure to the bleeding spot by putting a dressing inside the nose. Various types of dressings are available. If the nose is packed, admission to the hospital is sometimes necessary. Occasionally, the bleeding still fails to stop and then surgery is required to locate the bleeding vessel and deal with it under direct vision with the patient anesthetized. Rarely, the main blood vessel in the neck, the carotid artery, may have to be tied to stop bleeding.

HEARING LOSS

Hearing loss, or deafness, affects a large number of people, and becomes more common as people age. According to the National Institute on Deafness and Other Communication Disorders, 28 million Americans have hearing impairments.

What are the causes?

There are two types of hearing loss—sensorineural and conductive. Sensorineural hearing loss is when the inner ear is responsible for the deafness. The cochlea or the pathways from the cochlea to the brain are affected. The deafness may be present from birth or may be acquired later in life. Some infections such as meningitis, measles, and mumps can cause deafness, as can a skull fracture. The hearing loss of old age is sensorineural (p. 146).

Conductive deafness is when sound cannot reach the inner ear (cochlea) because of disease or blockage in the middle ear or ear canal. Causes include wax, glue ear (p. 144), and otosclerosis (p. 145).

How is it diagnosed?

Hearing loss is measured with a hearing test called audiometry (p. 108). To distinguish between the two types of deafness, the test is performed using headphones and a bone vibrator placed behind the ear. If the hearing loss is conductive, the sounds will be heard better with the bone vibrator than the headphones.

What are the treatment options?

Sensorineural hearing loss can be helped by amplifying residual hearing with a hearing aid. Many types of hearing aids are commercially available. For the profoundly deaf, a cochlear implant may be offered after careful assessment. Conductive hearing loss is dealt with by treating the underlying cause where possible, for example ear tube insertion for glue ear. Where treatment of the underlying condition is not possible or appropriate, a hearing aid can be worn with good effect.

What is the outlook?

This depends to an extent on the cause of the hearing loss, but hearing aid technology is improving all the time, with smaller and more sophisticated models coming onto the market. Many more profoundly deaf people are benefiting from cochlear implant surgery, and surgery for conductive hearing loss has been refined over the years. Screening of newborn babies for hearing ability can detect congenital hearing problems as soon as possible so that early treatment can be introduced to prevent delay in speech and language development.

Babies with hearing problems who receive hearing aids, visual and hearing stimulation, and who start learning to sign by the age of six months are likely to develop good communication skills.

INFECTIOUS MONONUCLEOSIS

Commonly known as glandular fever, this is an infection caused by a virus.

What is the cause?

Infectious mononucleosis (mono) is caused by the Epstein-Barr virus. The virus is passed from person to person in saliva, which is why the illness is also known as the "kissing disease." It is most common in adolescents or young adults, but can occur in children and the middle aged.

What are the symptoms?

Some patients may be infected without showing any signs of illness. The classic symptoms, however, are

- sore throat, which may be severe enough to prevent swallowing of saliva, and occasionally difficulty in breathing may occur;
- fever;
- swelling of glands in the neck and sometimes elsewhere in the body;
- lethargy and a general feeling of malaise;
- some swelling around the eyes, and a possible rash (the rash may be part of the disease, but can also occur if a patient with mono is prescribed the antibiotic ampicillin); and
- possible enlargement of the liver and spleen; a small number of patients develop jaundice.

How is it diagnosed?

A blood test can show whether the symptoms are caused by infectious mononucleosis.

What are the treatment options?

The viral infection must run its course, but symptoms can be relieved. The sore throat will respond to simple analgesics, such as acetaminophen or ibuprofen, and these will also help with any fever. Plenty of fluids should be taken. If the patient cannot swallow fluids, he or she may need to be admitted to the hospital for rehydration using an intravenous infusion (IV). Admission is also advised if there are breathing difficulties, and some patients may be given steroids while in the hospital to treat this. It is usually advisable to avoid contact sports for about a month if there has been enlargement of the spleen, so that it doesn't rupture.

What is the outlook?

The infection usually lasts for 1 to 2 weeks but is often followed by some months of tiredness before complete recovery. Full activity should be encouraged as early as possible. About 1 in 2000 affected people develop a chronic or recurrent form that may last for several months.

LABYRINTHITIS

An inflammation of the inner ear leading to balance problems or dizziness.

What are the causes?

Infection of the inner ear is commonly caused by a viral infection but can occur following a bacterial infection of the middle ear (see Otitis Media, p. 144).

What are the symptoms?

- Viral labyrinthitis often starts with a viral illness: The patient feels unwell and has flulike symptoms.
- This is followed by the onset of sudden severe dizziness associated with nausea and vomiting. The vertigo may be so severe that the patient can only lie still.

- The eyes dart rapidly from side to side; this is known as nystagmus (p. 109).
- As the condition settles down, the dizziness starts to get better, but there may be residual feelings of unsteadiness when moving the head for some weeks or months.

How is it diagnosed?

Because this complaint is thought to be due to a viral infection, in most cases the diagnosis is made on history and examination. The ears are examined to ensure that there is no middle ear infection present to cause the inner ear inflammation, and if the history suggests a viral infection and the ears look healthy, no further investigation is required. If the dizziness does not seem to improve as expected—the condition usually resolves over days and weeks—other causes need to be sought.

What are the treatment options?

With time, the brain starts to compensate for the dizziness, which gradually gets better. The worst of the illness is usually over within a few days, but residual

EXPERIENCING AN INNER EAR INFECTION

I had had a cold for a few days before the dizziness started. It came on suddenly out of the blue. The room started spinning and I couldn't focus—my eyes felt like they were jumping around. I thought I was going to faint and had to lie down. Then I felt sick and started to vomit.

My husband took me to an ENT office. After asking me how it had started and checking my ears, the doctor said it was probably a viral infection of the inner ear and gave me an injection to help the dizziness and sickness. I went home and lay down and within an hour I began to feel better. The sickness stopped and the dizziness was better as long as I lay still. The doctor, however, had urged me to get out of bed and move around because it would help my brain to start compensating for the upset to my balance, so I did this the next day. For some weeks, if I turned my head quickly, the dizziness returned for a few minutes, but this slowly got better and after about six weeks I was back to normal.

unsteadiness and feelings of dizziness with certain movements can take weeks or even months to settle completely. During the worst of the infection, medication such as prochlorperazine can help to suppress any dizziness and feeling of nausea. Any residual imbalance or dizziness may be helped by exercises that encourage the brain to adapt to the changes caused by the infection in the inner ear. These are known as Cawthorne–Cooksey, or vestibular rehabilitation, exercises (p. 76).

What is the outlook?

Nearly all cases resolve completely in time. If this does not happen, further investigation may be required to rule out other causes of balance problems such as Meniere's disease (p. 140).

LARYNGITIS

Inflammation of the larynx, the part of the throat involved with speaking.

What are the causes?

- Acute laryngitis is commonly caused by a viral infection or overuse of the voice, for example too much shouting at a football game.
- Chronic laryngitis is likely to be associated with smoking, excess alcohol consumption, acid reflux disease, or long-term voice overuse by people such as lawyers, teachers, and singers, people who work in noisy environments, or even children who scream excessively.

What are the symptoms?

- Acute laryngitis may be associated with a viral upper respiratory tract infection, such as the common cold, with all the associated symptoms. The throat feels sore and the voice starts to become croaky or husky. If the voice is not rested at this stage, it may disappear altogether for a while.
- Chronic laryngitis shares many of the symptoms of acute laryngitis but often without pain.

How is it diagnosed?

Most cases of acute laryngitis get better very quickly without needing any treatment from a doctor. If seen by a doctor, the diagnosis is usually made on the history and, if necessary, by examining the larynx with a mirror or endoscope. The vocal cords will appear reddened and swollen, and other areas of the larynx may be inflamed.

Any hoarseness that does not resolve within 4–6 weeks needs further investigation to rule out cancer of the larynx (p. 135), especially in high-risk groups such as smokers.

What are the treatment options?
- Acute laryngitis usually gets better without specific treatment because it is usually caused by a viral infection or short-term voice abuse. Most cases respond to simple measures such as resting the voice, drinking plenty of fluids, using a cool humidifier, and simple analgesia for the sore throat.
- Chronic laryngitis, if not a cancer symptom, will usually get better if smoking ceases and measures as for acute laryngitis are taken. If voice misuse is a factor, speech therapy may be helpful. Occasionally, if the vocal cords have become very swollen, surgery may be helpful to reduce the swelling and so improve the voice. Treatment for acid reflux will also reduce swelling.

LARYNGOMALACIA
A condition seen in newborn babies in which the tissues of the larynx are floppy, causing noisy breathing.

What are the causes?
The laryngeal tissues are floppy at birth because of immaturity of the supporting cartilage.

What are the symptoms?
The baby develops noisy or squeaky breathing, usually on breathing in, within an hour or two or up to several weeks after birth. The symptoms may be worsened by
- feeding;
- lying on the back;
- infections such as colds;
- agitation.

Rarely, the condition may obstruct breathing.

How is it diagnosed?
If symptoms are mild and there is no interference with feeding, no further investigation is required, and the child merely needs checking at the ENT office at regular intervals until he or she grows out of the condition.

If the symptoms are more severe or interfere with feeding, the larynx needs to be examined. It is sometimes possible to do this in the ENT office with a very fine flexible endoscope if the baby is cooperative, but more usually a general anesthetic is required.

What are the treatment options?
- Laryngomalacia gets better as the baby gets older and the cartilage supporting the larynx matures. For most children, no treatment is necessary.
- If the condition is severe, it can interfere with feeding, because the baby finds it difficult to breathe and feed at the same time. The child may fail to gain weight and become undernourished. In such cases, and those in which the breathing is severely affected, the larynx is usually examined under a general anesthetic. This will confirm the diagnosis and make sure that there is no other reason for the problems encountered. At the same time, any surplus tissue that may be getting in the way of breathing can be removed. In very severe cases, in which the baby is struggling to breathe adequately, a tracheostomy (p. 129) may be necessary as a temporary measure until the condition starts to resolve.

What is the outlook?
The symptoms gradually improve with time. It can sometimes take a few years for the larynx to become firm enough to resist collapse on breathing in, but all children will grow out of the condition.

MENIERE'S DISEASE
First described in 1861 by Prosper Meniere, this condition of the inner ear is characterized by vertigo (dizziness), tinnitus, and deafness.

What is the cause?
It is thought to be caused by a sudden increase in the volume of fluid called endolymph in the inner ear. The cause of this increase is unknown but is being actively researched. The condition is more common in middle age and appears to occur equally among women and men. There is often a history of migraines in the family, but the link is uncertain.

What are the symptoms?
The main feature of Meniere's disease is that it occurs in episodes, and between them, sufferers are often well with few symptoms. The main symptoms include the following:
- Dizziness (vertigo) Attacks vary in frequency, with some patients having just one or two per year and others having more frequent episodes. The dizziness may last minutes or hours, with some patients experiencing nausea and vomiting during an attack. After an attack has finished, the sufferer may feel unwell for several days.

- **Tinnitus** A ringing or buzzing noise in the ear is often noticed during an attack. In the early stages of the disease, the tinnitus disappears completely between attacks, but as time goes by it can become constant.
- **Hearing loss** This is associated with the dizzy spells. At first it may be described as a feeling of fullness or blockage in the ear that gets better as the attack subsides, but as the attacks continue, the hearing recovers to a lesser degree after each attack, until a permanent sensorineural hearing loss (p. 137) is experienced.

How is it diagnosed?

In the early stages, there may be little to find, because all returns to normal between attacks. Patients are usually seen at an ENT office between attacks, and various tests are performed.

- **Hearing test** This is performed in all cases of suspected Meniere's disease and may show evidence of a sensorineural hearing loss. If the test is repeated at intervals between attacks, it may show the fluctuation of the hearing and eventually the gradual worsening and permanent hearing loss. Usually, only one ear is affected, although about one third of patients eventually go on to develop disease in the second ear.
- **Tests of vestibular function** These record the function of the part of the inner ear responsible for balance—this is the part responsible for the dizziness experienced by patients. A number of tests are available, including a caloric test and electrocochleography or an MRI scan. It may sometimes be necessary to rule out the possibility of an acoustic neuroma (p. 134) in a patient with hearing loss in one ear only before assuming it is due to Meniere's disease.

What are the treatment options?

Treatment may be medical or surgical, and the simplest treatments are usually tried first.

Initially, most patients are treated medically. Lifestyle measures include quitting smoking, which will improve blood flow to the nerve endings of the inner ear; reducing the intake of salt to decrease the accumulation of fluid in the inner ear; and eliminating caffeine to avoid excess stimulation of the nerve endings. Drugs used to treat the attacks as they occur include diphenhydinate and meclizine; these will reduce the sickness associated with an attack, as well as alleviate the dizziness. Diuretics have also been tried, with varying success. Betahistine is common in other countries, including Canada and the U.K. It has not yet been approved by the FDA, so it is not commercially available in the United States.

A procedure known as intratympanic gentamicin, in which an antibiotic called gentamicin is injected through the eardrum, can be carried out on an outpatient basis. When used in doses to fight infection elsewhere in the body, this antibiotic can have the unfortunate side effect of damaging the inner ear, an effect that is exploited in this situation. The drug is put into the middle ear through the drum, with the intention of damaging the part of the inner ear responsible for balance and stopping the dizzy spells. The disadvantage of this treatment is that it can also destroy hearing in that ear. However, for those experiencing frequent severe attacks of dizziness that are very disabling, this may be a price worth paying.

Various techniques have been tried over the years to cure the condition with surgery. The simplest procedure is the insertion of an ear tube (p. 120). There is no good explanation as to why this should work—some have even claimed it is due to the placebo effect—but in some patients the procedure brings relief of symptoms.

The main surgical treatment for Meniere's disease is endolymphatic saccus decompression. The sac is part of the inner ear and is normally covered by the bone of the skull. By opening up the area behind the ear (known as the mastoid bone) the saccus is exposed, and it is thought that this enables it to expand freely when the fluid in the inner ear increases during an attack.

A more radical operation is one that cuts the nerve running from the balance apparatus to the brain. This requires the skull to be opened and hence carries more risk of complications, but it does appear to relieve symptoms. If there is little useful hearing left in the affected ear, a labyrinthectomy may be carried out to cure the symptoms, but this will destroy both the inner ear and any hearing.

What is the outlook?

In many cases, the disease seems to burn itself out after a number of years. The dizzy attacks cease and the hearing stops deteriorating, although it does not recover. The tinnitus may also remain. Prior to reaching this stage, many cases are well controlled by medication. Research continues into this distressing condition.

About 90 percent of patients report relief of symptoms of Meniere's disease after endolymphatic saccus decompression, but only 60 percent claim continued relief after five years.

MOTION SICKNESS
A feeling of nausea that may lead to actual vomiting, usually experienced while traveling.

What are the causes?
The balance part of the inner ear is very sensitive to changes in position. In some people, it is so sensitive that even minor frequent changes, such as those experienced when traveling in a car, is enough to confuse the brain. So many different signals are received in rapid succession that the brain can no longer tell which way up the body is or which way it is facing. This leads to the stimulation of various receptors that in turn leads to feelings of sickness and can, in extremes, cause vomiting.

What are the treatment options?
Various medications are available for motion sickness. Some, such as scopolamine, prevent the onset of symptoms if taken in advance. Antihistamines such as diphenhydrinate, also taken before traveling, can help to stave off sickness and have fewer side effects, but they are a little less effective. These drugs all work by suppressing the balance mechanism of the inner ear and the part of the brain responsible for vomiting.

Describing ENT symptoms

When describing symptoms, it will help your doctor to help you if you can be precise about them. A clear history will enable the doctor to make a final diagnosis and prescribe appropriate medication. Note such factors as these:

- *Does dizziness feel like the room spinning or just a lightheaded feeling? Does it happen only with certain movements of the head or can it come on even when sitting still?*

- *Does motion sickness come on with every journey, only on certain types of transportation, or at other times, such as at the movies?*

- *Are nosebleeds common, infrequent, or only happen after a cold or other infection?*

- *Is snoring an every-night occurrence or does it only happen after drinking alcohol late?*

What is the outlook?
Adaptation does occur in people who are in a prolonged situation that induces motion sickness, such as on a ship. Many young sailors suffer from sickness on a first long sea voyage, but for most, the sickness gradually settles until they have no further problems.

NASAL POLYPOSIS
A condition in which the membrane lining the nasal cavity becomes thickened and produces swellings.

When the lining of the nose becomes inflamed, it becomes swollen. If this swelling continues untreated, the lining becomes more and more swollen and areas fill with fluid. These gelatinous sacs on the nasal or sinus lining are called polyps (a swelling with a stalk).

What are the causes?
The initial inflammation may be triggered by a number of factors, including chronic infection and allergy. There are certain groups of patients, such as people with asthma, in whom polyps are more likely to form, particularly if they are allergic to aspirin.

What are the symptoms?
Although they are small, the polyps may not show any symptoms, although if associated with allergies, the symptoms may initially be put down to these. The most common complaints are of nasal obstruction and nasal speech. As the polyps enlarge, there may be a clear watery discharge from the nose. The sense of smell is often poor, and this affects the sense of taste. There is sometimes a headache and pressure across the face, and sinusitis may occur. If ignored for a long time, the polyps can become so large that they hang out of the nose and cause it to widen.

How is it diagnosed?
It is easy to see even small polyps using an endoscope. If surgery is necessary, a CT scan is sometimes obtained to help plan the procedure, or if there are polyps in only one side of the nose, to rule out a tumor. Other tests relate to the underlying causes, such as skin testing for allergies.

What are the treatment options?
Unless the polyps are very large, the first choice for the majority of cases is medical treatment. This consists of sprays or drops into the nose that contain a small dose of

a steroid that acts on the polyps directly to reduce the inflammation and cause them to shrink. Very little of the steroid administered in this way is absorbed into the body, so the usual side effects associated with steroid use are rarely encountered. Occasionally, a short course of steroid tablets may be used to get things under control.

Surgery is appropriate in those cases where the polyps are large or if sinusitis (p. 150) is an associated problem. Most surgery is performed using an endoscope, but other types of surgery are occasionally used to treat severe cases. After surgery, most patients need medical treatment to help prevent recurrence of the polyps.

What is the outlook?
For some patients, particularly those with asthma or an aspirin allergy, the polyps will keep coming back. It is thought that prolonged treatment with drops or sprays helps increase the time between recurrences, but it may not prevent them completely. Nasal polyposis is an area of much ongoing research, and the pathways involved in inflammation are constantly being looked at to develop new drugs that may suppress the underlying background of inflammation in patients with polyps.

Ongoing research into drugs to combat nasal polyps may mean that one day most patients will be treated solely with drugs and surgery will become rare.

OBSTRUCTIVE SLEEP APNEA (OSA)
A condition in which breathing is obstructed during sleep to the extent that breathing stops and the sufferer awakes.

Obstructive sleep apnea can affect adults and children. It is more common in adult males than in females and affects younger children rather than older.

What are the causes?
In adults, the airway becomes obstructed during sleep by the collapse of the soft tissues from the nose to the voice box. In children, obstruction is usually caused by the relatively large size of the adenoids and tonsils. As the person breathes in, the tissues cause complete obstruction of the airway, and no air is actually drawn in. In adults, certain factors make sleep apnea more likely. These include
- obesity;
- alcohol consumption;
- age—the condition is more common as age increases; and
- gender—it is more common in males.

What are the symptoms?
The patient's history is very important, in particular that from the sleeping partner or parent. It can be very frightening for the onlooker to see a person struggling for breath, and many report waking the sufferer at intervals to make him or her breathe. If left alone, the affected person will breathe spontaneously as his or her level of consciousness rises because of the lowered oxygen level and increased carbon dioxide in the blood. The resulting interrupted sleep can lead to a number of symptoms during the day.
- **Daytime sleepiness** This may be responsible for a number of road accidents caused by people falling asleep while driving. Children may be miserable during the day and need more naps than usual.
- **Morning headaches** These may be caused by the raised level of carbon dioxide in the blood and lack of oxygen.
- **Lack of concentration**
- **Impotence**

How is it diagnosed?
To make a diagnosis, a sleep study must be undertaken. The subject is attached to monitors while sleeping. These record, among other things, periods of obstruction when no air passes, the level of oxygen in the blood, blood pressure, and heart rate. Admission to hospital overnight is usual. Some specialists perform a sleep nasoendoscopy, giving the patient a drug to induce sleep and inserting an endoscope through the nose to examine the entire larynx.

How is it treated?
Losing weight and reducing alcohol consumption are recommended for all adults. For severe sleep apnea, continuous positive airway pressure (CPAP) is the treatment of choice. This involves wearing a mask at night that provides air at a pressure that keeps the airway open. Surgery may also be an option. In children, the removal of the adenoids and tonsils is recommended. Less severe OSA may be managed by a mandibular advancement splint—a type of gum shield worn at night that opens the airway.

OTITIS EXTERNA
Infection or inflammation of the ear canal.

What are the causes?
Otitis externa may be acute or chronic. The chronic cases tend to be associated with skin problems, such as eczema, which predisposes the skin of the ear canal to infection,

particularly when wet. Acute infections are often secondary to other factors, such as trauma to the ear canal from the use of cotton swabs or fingernails for cleaning the ear or water in the ear when swimming or bathing. The infection may be bacterial and sometimes fungal.

What are the symptoms?
Symptoms include pain, swelling of the ear canal or whole ear, discharge from the ear, and itching.

How is it diagnosed?
Otitis externa is diagnosed with patient history and examination. In the event of no response to the prescribed treatment, a sample may be taken from the ear canal to see which microorganisms are responsible for the infection.

How is it treated?
Discharge in the ear canal should be cleaned prior to using any drops. If the ear canal is swollen, a dressing in the canal may be required, because drops may not reach the deeper parts of the canal. Eardrops containing antibiotics and steroids to reduce the swelling are usually prescribed.

In severe cases, with spread of infection to the whole ear or face, admission to the hospital for intravenous antibiotics may be advised. For chronic eczema of the ear canal, steroid eardrops and creams may be recommended. In all cases, it is important to keep water out of the ears. Generally, cleaning the ears with cotton swabs or any other implement is not recommended.

OTITIS MEDIA
An inflammation of the middle ear.

The middle ear is the space behind the eardrum, which can become inflamed during an infection.

What are the causes?
Otitis media may be acute or chronic. Acute otitis media is often associated with upper respiratory tract infections. It is caused by infection of the middle ear from bacteria reaching the middle ear through the eustachian tube. It is more common in young children. Most children have frequent colds, and the adenoids may be enlarged, causing blockage of the eustachian tube.

Chronic otitis media, or otitis media with effusion, is also known as glue ear. The fundamental problem here is eustachian tube dysfunction. The pressure behind the eardrum is unable to equalize, because air cannot get up the tube. Consequently, the pressure in the middle ear falls. This causes inflammation of the middle ear lining, and fluid is produced that fills the middle ear space. The eustachian tube may be functioning poorly because of adenoidal hypertrophy, immaturity, or problems such as a cleft palate and tumor in the back of the nose.

What are the symptoms?
Acute otitis media causes pain, fever, and deafness. If untreated, the eardrum may burst: This relieves the pain, but the fluid then leaks from the ear. Chronic otitis media, or glue ear, is usually characterized by hearing loss. Because the fluid has built up gradually, it is usually painless unless infected.

How is it diagnosed?
Examination of the ear reveals the presence of fluid behind the eardrum, and a hearing test confirms a conductive hearing loss. If the eardrum is not moving due to fluid behind it, the tympanometry test (p. 108) will produce a flat tracing.

What are the treatment options?
Acute otitis media will often get better within 24 hours without treatment. If not, it responds well to antibiotics. These will usually be taken orally, but if it is felt that the infection has spread into the mastoid bone, a condition known as mastoiditis, intravenous antibiotics are

Why do some children with middle ear infection have their adenoids removed?

The adenoids are lumps of lymphoid tissue similar to the tonsils found at the back of the nose. They tend to be biggest between the ages of three and eight years and then shrink in size. Because of their position at the back of the nose, it is thought that they can cause blockage of the eustachian tube and therefore play a role in the formation of middle ear infection and acute otitis media. There is still much debate as to whether removal has much effect on the control of otitis media, however. Some studies show a significant improvement, especially in older children.

ASK THE EXPERT

required. Chronic otitis media, or glue ear, is often a self-limiting condition, especially in children. There is, therefore, a good case for watching and waiting. Most specialists recommend review after three months, because some children get better without treatment during that period.

Further treatment is usually recommended in the following situations:
- Persistent deafness causing behavioral problems or difficulties at school.
- When the eardrum is becoming unhealthy and is in danger of collapsing. This can be a precursor to the formation of a benign tumor of the middle ear known as a cholesteatoma.

For chronic otitis media, the usual treatment is the insertion of a ventilation tube. The adenoids may sometimes be removed.

If the main problem is hearing loss and the parents are against surgical intervention, a hearing aid can be useful. In adults with glue ear on one side only, tests should be done to exclude a tumor at the back of the nose when the ear tube is inserted.

What is the outlook?
The natural history of both acute and chronic otitis media is one of spontaneous improvement. Most children will grow out of the problem, so intervention depends upon the severity of the symptoms. If tubes are inserted, they usually expel themselves after about a year, and only one quarter of children will need another set.

OTOSCLEROSIS
The formation of new bone in the middle ear that interferes with the conduction of sound to the cochlea.

Otosclerosis is an inherited disease in which abnormal bone grows in the middle ear. This results in deafness because the small bones of the middle ear (ossicles) become fixed and so are unable to conduct sound from the eardrum to the inner ear efficiently. Occasionally, the inner ear is also involved.

What are the symptoms?
Deafness is the primary symptom and tends to occur before the age of 30. It particularly affects women. Many patients also suffer with tinnitus (p. 152), especially if the inner ear is involved.

How is it diagnosed?
A hearing test typically shows a marked deafness due to poor conduction of sound from the outside world to the inner ear. If the inner ear is involved, there is an additional sensory element to the hearing loss.

What are the treatment options?
Some people with mild otosclerosis do not require treatment. However, in those with significant deafness, the two main options are a hearing aid or surgery. A hearing aid is simple, effective, and risk-free but has the obvious disadvantage of being visible behind and within the ear. The operation—called a stapedectomy—involves drilling a tiny 0.02-inch wide hole in the stapes and bypassing the fixed segment by inserting a piston. The operation is successful in more than 90 percent of cases, but certain risks are associated with it. In particular, there is a 1 percent chance of losing the hearing in that ear. Some patients suffer with vertigo, but this resolves after a few days.

Up to 10 percent of the Caucasion population is thought to be affected by otosclerosis to some degree, although only 1 percent suffers from footplate otosclerosis. Up to 70 percent have hearing loss in both ears.

PHARYNGITIS
Inflammation of the lining of either the throat or the pharynx.

Pharyngitis is very common and may be acute or chronic. The acute form is probably the most common cause of "sore throats" in adults.

What are the causes?
Acute pharyngitis is most commonly caused by a viral infection, but it can be bacterial in origin. In contrast, the chronic form of the disease may be caused by irritation by cigarette smoke or alcohol. It may also follow contact with infected mucus in a patient with sinusitis, or it may result from acid reflux from the stomach. In many patients, no cause can be identified. A chronic sore throat may be a symptom of malignancy, so a sore throat that lasts for more than four weeks should be seen by an ENT specialist.

What are the symptoms?
Both acute and chronic pharyngitis are characterized by a sore throat. In addition, acute pharyngitis is often associated with a multitude of other symptoms depending

on which other areas are affected. There is often a fever with general malaise and there may be a runny or stuffy nose, hoarseness if the larynx is affected, or cough if the lungs are affected. In contrast, chronic pharyngitis often has no symptoms except a sore throat. However, there may be symptoms of the underlying condition, for example of sinusitis or of gastroesophageal reflux.

How is it diagnosed?
The symptoms are the most important aid to diagnosis, but examination may show an inflamed pharynx with infected mucus present. The examination may not show anything specific in those with chronic pharyngitis.

What are the treatment options?
Acute pharyngitis is self-limiting and usually resolves after 4 to 5 days. Treatment involves pain relief and plenty of fluids. Antibiotics are rarely required, because the underlying cause is usually viral. Treatment of chronic pharyngitis depends on the underlying cause. If smoking or alcohol consumption is a contributing factor, it should be stopped. Sinusitis or gastroesophageal reflux are treated as appropriate. Examination of the pharynx, under anesthetic if necessary, should be carried out in selected cases to make sure there is not an underlying malignancy.

HELP YOUR DOCTOR HELP YOU

Describing a sore throat
Your doctor needs to know the following about a sore throat in order to reach a diagnosis and recommend appropriate treatment.

- *How long the sore throat has persisted, whether you have had a sore throat before, and whether family members also have sore throats or have had them recently.*

- *Whether the pain is worse at night or in the morning or if it prevents you from sleeping.*

- *Does anything relieve it (such as a warm drink or painkillers) or make it worse (such as swallowing or breathing through the mouth)?*

- *Whether your voice is affected; has it almost gone or is it simply hoarse?*

- *Is the sore throat getting better or worse, or is it about the same?*

PRESBYCUSIS
Age-related hearing loss.

It is an inevitability that our hearing deteriorates as we get older. This can cause considerable functional impairment in the elderly person, who may also have other medical problems to contend with.

What is the cause?
The cause of presbycusis is not known, but the condition involves a deterioration in the number of nerve fibers supplying the cochlea and in the hair cells responsible for detecting sound. Thus, the quality of the information passing to the brain from the inner ear deteriorates.

What are the symptoms?
Deterioration of hearing in both ears is the primary symptom. A loss of the ability to discriminate between words makes understanding speech a problem, especially in noisy environments. There may also be distortion of sounds. The ear looks normal when examined.

How is it diagnosed?
A hearing test confirms the diagnosis in conjunction with a thorough medical history. There is, typically, a particular loss of hearing of high frequencies.

What are the treatment options?
Early presbycusis may not require any treatment except reassurance that there is no underlying problem with the ears. As the process progresses and the hearing loss becomes severe, the best method of treatment is a hearing aid. There is no surgical method of improving the hearing of people with this condition.

What is the outlook?
The deterioration is often progressive and eventually those who are worst affected can become profoundly deaf. There is a wide spectrum of severity, however, and many people only experience mild degrees of presbycusis.

QUINSY
An abscess next to the tonsil following acute tonsillitis.

Tonsillar infection is very common and in the most severe cases can result in the formation of pus and the development of an abscess in the tissues around the tonsil, hence its alternative name of peritonsillar abscess. This often makes the symptoms much more severe. It tends to affect young adults and is rare in children.

What are the causes?
The cause is the same as that for tonsillitis: an acute bacterial infection. The reason why some people develop an abscess and others do not is not understood.

What are the symptoms?
Sore throat, difficulty swallowing, and fever are present, as they are for tonsillitis. However, the pain may be more severe, particularly on the affected side. It may be difficult to open the mouth because the abscess causes inflammation of the muscles involved in opening the mouth and there is often a hot potato quality to the voice caused by the swelling in the throat. If it is not treated, the swelling can affect breathing and can therefore be life-threatening.

How is it diagnosed?
The typical appearance in the throat is of a striking swelling in the area just above the upper part of the affected tonsil. The presence of pus when the abscess is opened confirms the diagnosis.

What are the treatment options?
Pain relief and antibiotics are an important part of treating this problem. However, like any abscess, it will rarely resolve when there is still a collection of pus present. Thus, the abscess must be drained. Traditionally, after anesthetizing the area, the abscess was incised using a knife. More recently, ENT surgeons have favored removing the pus using a needle and syringe. This is often less painful and less traumatic to the lining of the throat.

What is the outlook?
The peritonsillar infection usually resolves quickly once the abscess is drained. Those who experience more than one episode of quinsy are usually advised to undergo tonsillectomy in order to prevent further problems.

RHINITIS
Inflammation of the membranes lining the nose.

Rhinitis is a very common condition that affects one in six people and its incidence is increasing. The lining of the nose is continuous with that of the sinuses and inflammation in the nose goes hand in hand with inflammation of the sinuses. Rhinitis is also frequently associated with asthma.

What are the causes?
Rhinitis may be part of a viral upper respiratory tract infection—"the common cold"— or it may be secondary to a bacterial infection, as with acute sinusitis. There is also evidence that reactions to fungus may be responsible for some cases of rhinitis. Other forms of the disease are caused by allergy and there are many possible allergens. The most common is pollen and this constitutes "hay fever." Other common allergens include dust, dust mites, feathers, and animal fur. The inflammation may also be part of a more generalized disease such as cystic fibrosis or rheumatoid arthritis. In some people, there is no obvious cause.

What are the symptoms?
People suffering with this condition may experience a number of symptoms. There may be nasal blockage, runny nose, mucus dripping down the back of the nose, sneezing, or nasal itching. Secondary symptoms such as facial pain and loss of the sense of smell may also occur.

How is it diagnosed?
The diagnosis is based on the symptoms and confirmed by clinical examination. The lining of the nose typically looks swollen and inflamed and there is usually mucus within the nose that may be watery in the case of allergy-induced rhinitis or green in the case of bacterial infection. Skin prick allergy tests confirm whether or not there is an allergic element.

A number of more specialized tests are available to help diagnose some of the rarer causes of the disease, and in those people who do not respond to treatment, a CT scan of the sinuses may be required.

What are the treatment options?
This depends on the cause of the problem. For those with allergic rhinitis, one of the most important aspects of treatment is advice on avoiding the allergen that is causing it. Because there is no cure for this condition, the other arm of treatment is symptomatic relief. Several effective medications are available, the mainstay of treatment being topical steroid nasal sprays. These generally have very low absorption rates and are, therefore, rarely associated with side effects, although dryness and occasional nosebleeds can occur.

In those with severe and resistant symptoms, a course of oral steroids can be prescribed. For those people suffering with sneezing, itching, or a runny nose, oral antihistamines can be used. There is also a topical preparation available for external use. Decongestants can be used temporarily but tend to make the symptoms worse if used over a prolonged period.

Rhinitis is the most common chronic illness of human beings.

What is the outlook?
There is no cure for most forms of rhinitis, but in most cases the symptoms can be effectively controlled with the right advice and medication. Those who have persistent problems despite these measures may benefit from investigation of their sinuses. This is carried out by a endoscopic technique and if necessary by CT scanning.

RUPTURED EARDRUM
A hole that develops in the eardrum.

Rupture, or perforation, of the eardrum can occur as a result of middle ear infection, injury, or following surgery on the ear. Repeated tube insertion (p. 120) can result in persistent perforation. In most cases, the eardrum heals completely, but occasionally the process is incomplete and the individual is left with a hole in the drum.

What are the symptoms?
If the perforation is traumatic, there will be pain, deafness, and often a bloody discharge from the ear. If there is injury to the inner ear as well, in a skull fracture for example, there may be dizziness and deafness. If the rupture is the result of infection, the symptoms will include fever and general malaise, together with deafness and a yellow or green discharge from the ear. Once the acute event is over, there may be no symptoms. In fact, some people will have a perforated eardrum and not even be aware of it. In those who do have symptoms, the most common are deafness and recurrent infections, particularly after swimming or bathing in contaminated water.

How is it diagnosed?
The diagnosis is made by examining the ear. The hole is usually clearly visible, and the structures of the middle ear can often be seen, too. Tests of the functioning of the middle ear (tympanometry, p. 108) can also be used to confirm the diagnosis.

SUFFERING A RUPTURED EARDRUM

I've been diving for several years now, and I rarely have any problems with my ears. Last summer, though, on a diving excursion, I mistimed my ascent and ended up rupturing my right eardrum. It was really painful at first, then after a few hours it just ached. I also had some bleeding from the ear.

More worrisome than these symptoms, however, was the hearing loss. I went deaf and developed a ringing in my ear. The local doctor confirmed that I'd ruptured the eardrum and forbade me from diving until I'd had the ear checked by a specialist.

Over the next few days, the pain settled down and the ringing went away, much to my relief. My hearing also came back, and by the time I got back home and saw the specialist, the hole had healed up. The specialist explained that most ruptures heal by themselves. I'm glad I didn't need surgery and will take even more care with my dives in future.

What are the treatment options?
Infection in the middle ear should be treated with oral or local antibiotics, although there is some concern that certain local antibiotics can damage the cochlea, resulting in further deafness. Traumatic perforations usually heal by themselves within two months, so a doctor will simply observe the drum during that time.

If a perforation is persistent, a number of options are available. No treatment is needed if the perforation is not causing problems, although patients are advised to keep the ear dry to avoid infection. If the only symptom is hearing loss, this can be overcome with a hearing aid. If there is recurrent infection, or significant hearing loss and the patient does not wish to have a hearing aid, surgical repair can be carried out. The basic principle is to cover the perforation with tissue from elsewhere in the body, often from the temple of the face. This acts as a scaffolding so that the remaining drum can heal and fill in the defect. The operation is successful in about 80 percent of cases.

SINGER'S (OR VOCAL) NODULES
Swellings or nodules that develop on the vocal cords as a result of poor voice habits.

Singer's nodes or vocal nodules are a common complaint and can occur in both children and adults. They tend to affect women more than men. They form as a result of overuse or misuse of the voice. Thus, those who sing, talk a lot, or frequently shout are most likely to develop a problem. A part of each side of the vocal cord becomes swollen because of the trauma and, if the misuse continues, the swollen area becomes scarred. Once this stage is reached, the damage is often irreversible.

What are the symptoms?
The voice becomes breathy, husky, and low pitched because the two sides of the vocal cords are no longer able to vibrate and come together effectively.

How is it diagnosed?
The definitive diagnosis is made by examining the voice box with a flexible endoscope. This allows identification of the nodules and exclusion of any other disease, such as a vocal cord paralysis or a malignancy. A more detailed examination of vocal cord function can be obtained using a special endoscope attached to a video camera that allows a real-time recording of vocal cord movements.

Are nodules on the vocal cords an early sign of throat cancer?

No—nodules are benign. They develop as a result of overuse or abuse of the voice and cause the vocal cords to swell and harden, which eventually results in hoarseness. Because hoarseness is also one of the symptoms of throat cancer, an ENT specialist may take a biopsy of any nodules to ensure that they are benign, but there is usually no cause for concern. Nodules respond best to voice rest and speech therapy to ensure that the poor habits that caused them are not continued. Some surgeons opt to remove nodules, but the available evidence suggests that without speech therapy to train a patient to use the voice wisely, nodules are likely to return.

ASK THE EXPERT

What are the treatment options?
The main aim of treatment is to reeducate the voice and correct the bad habits that have led to the formation of nodules. Exercises are recommended to reduce stress on the voice, eliminate the damaging habits, and teach the individual how to use his or her voice correctly. The majority of vocal nodules will resolve in this way. Complete voice rest can also be successful, but it is difficult to maintain for an adequate length of time and does not correct the underlying problem, so the nodules tend to recur once the patient starts using the voice again. Close examination of the voice box under a general anesthetic and removal of the nodules by microsurgery is sometimes necessary.

SINUSITIS
Inflammation of the sinuses.

In the majority of cases, inflammation of the sinuses goes hand in hand with inflammation of the nose. Hence, a more correct term for this disease is rhinosinusitis.

What are the causes?
As with rhinitis, there are many different causes of sinusitus. It may be allergic or infective in origin. Infection may be viral, as with the common cold, or bacterial. There is increasing evidence for a fungal cause in some cases. Any infection can be acute or chronic. Similarly, it may be secondary to a more generalized illness, such as cystic fibrosis, rheumatoid arthritis, or Wegener's granulomatosis.

What are the symptoms?
This depends on the cause, but typical symptoms are nasal blockage and a runny nose, which may be watery in allergic cases or thick and yellow or green in cases of infection. There is often mucus dripping into the throat from the back of the nose and facial pain due to pressure buildup in the sinuses. There may also be a loss of smell.

In severe infective cases, complications can develop. These include infection around the eye that can potentially damage vision, infection of the bone forming the walls of the sinuses, and spread of the infection to the brain or its coverings, resulting in meningitis or brain abscess.

How is it diagnosed?
The diagnosis is made with the patient's description of the symptoms and then confirmed by physical examination. The nasal lining is swollen and inflamed and there is a

discharge within the nose. In difficult cases, those that fail to respond to treatment or are suspected of having complications, a CT scan of the sinuses is obtained.

What are the treatment options?
The treatment depends on the underlying cause. Chronic inflammation caused by allergies should be treated in the same way as allergic rhinitis (p. 147) and includes avoiding allergens and using steroids inside the nose and oral anti-histamines. Bacterial rhinosinusitis is treated with oral antibiotics together with a short course of a decongestant followed by a steroid applied inside the nose. Viral rhinosinusitis requires only treatment of symptoms. Fungal sinusitis may require antifungal medications. If medical treatment fails, surgical drainage of the sinuses can be carried out, usually by endoscopic techniques.

What is the outlook?
Infective sinusitis can resolve completely with treatment. There is no cure for allergic rhinosinusitis, but in most patients good symptomatic relief can be obtained.

SNORING
Noise generated during sleep caused by partial obstruction of the upper airway.

The number of people who snore has probably risen over the past few decades as a result of an increase in the number of people who are overweight. This is perhaps perhaps the most common contributing factor. However, the number of people consulting their doctors and ENT specialists for the problem has risen even faster, which partly reflects increased awareness of the availability of treatments. Snoring itself often causes significant disturbance, particularly to partners. In a proportion of cases, it is associated with intermittent complete obstruction of the airway—obstructive sleep apnea, or OSA (p. 143).

What are the causes?
The noise of snoring occurs as a result of vibrations that develop between the soft palate or the walls of the pharynx. These are particularly likely to develop if the airway is narrowed for some reason. In adults, sites of narrowing include the nose, because of deviation of the nasal septum or rhinitis, and the throat, because of a floppy soft palate, bulky tongue, or generalized narrowing of the pharynx as a result of obesity. Alcohol abuse also predisposes people to snoring and OSA. In children, the adenoids and tonsils are proportionally larger than they are in adults. They can, therefore, cause narrowing of the airway and thus snoring and obstructive sleep apnea.

What are the symptoms?
Simple snorers usually have no other symptoms except snoring. It is their partners who suffer with lack of sleep, leading to tiredness, irritability, and loss of concentration the following day. The partner often resorts to sleeping in a separate room if possible, and in the most extreme cases, marital difficulties can arise. It is important to have the partner present when discussing the problem. In contrast, those suffering with obstructive sleep apnea themselves suffer from daytime tiredness, poor concentration, personality change, and increased risk of traffic accidents. The low oxygen level in the blood that results from OSA can cause high blood pressure, excessive strain on the heart, and an irregular heartbeat.

How is it diagnosed?
The most important aspects of diagnosis are to identify whether or not the snorer suffers with obstructive sleep apnea and the site from which the obstruction originates. A combination of the symptoms that the person describes and thorough clinical examination usually answers these questions. The nose and throat are examined with a flexible endoscope, and the patient's sleep patterns are assessed formally in an overnight sleep study.

Are all snorers at risk of obstructive sleep apnea?

Snoring is a very common problem that in itself causes more difficulties for the partner than it does for the snorer. It results from the vibration of two adjacent surfaces in the lining of the nose or throat and is more likely to occur if these structures are narrowed for some reason, for example, as a result of obesity. In more extreme cases, the throat can become temporarily blocked during sleep, resulting in sleep apnea. Not everyone who snores suffers with sleep apnea, but many snorers are at risk for developing the problem, especially those who are overweight.

ASK THE EXPERT

Laser-assisted uvulopalatoplasty

Developed in France in the early 1990s, laser-assisted uvulopalatoplasty is carried out to reduce snoring and sleep apnea. The technique involves the removal by laser of part of the uvula and back of the soft palate to widen the airway. Usually only one session of treatment is needed. The laser cuts down on bleeding and on postoperative pain, but studies suggest mixed results. Some document improvements in snoring in up to 80 percent of patients. The success rate depends on correct evaluation to identify only palatal snorers.

What are the treatment options?

People with simple snoring problems do not necessarily require any medical treatment. Reassurance that there is no serious underlying pathological cause, with appropriate weight loss and reduction of alcohol consumption, are often all that is required. If the nose is responsible for the obstruction, septal deviation can be surgically corrected and rhinitis can be treated. If the problem is caused by the soft palate, surgical shortening of the uvula or stiffening of the palate by excision of excess tissue can be performed.

A bulky tongue base can be treated using a special splint—a device similar to braces—at night to bring the jaw forward and increase the volume of the airway. Surgery to reduce tongue size to prevent prolapse is also an option. If the obstruction originates in the throat, the airways can be kept open overnight by increasing the pressure inside the throat using a special mask (continuous positive airway pressure). This is often effective, but many people find the mask uncomfortable. In the most extreme cases of obstructive sleep apnea, a tracheotomy (p. 129) can be lifesaving. In children, an adenoidectomy or tonsillectomy is usually successful in resolving the problem.

STRIDOR

Noisy breathing resulting from partial obstruction of the airway at or below the level of the voice box.

Stridor is often confused with the wheeze that is symptomatic of asthma. The main difference between them, however, is that stridor tends to be a difficulty with breathing in, whereas the wheeze from asthma tends to be a difficulty with breathing out. A third condition, stertor, is noisy breathing resulting from partial obstruction of the airway above the larynx, for example by large tonsils.

What are the causes?

The causes of stridor can be divided into problems that the individual was born with (congenital) and those that are acquired through some event or disease process. Congenital problems include
- weakness of the structure of the voice box or trachea, which results in collapse;
- laryngotracheomalacia—congenital narrowing of the voice box or trachea (stenosis); and
- benign tumors of the airway such as hemangiomata.

Acquired causes include
- injury from thermal or chemical burns or direct trauma;
- inflammation as a result of infection or other inflammatory condition;
- inhaled foreign bodies within the airway;
- paralysis of one or both of the vocal cords;
- swelling within the airway following an allergic reaction;
- narrowing of the airway caused by a tumor; and
- narrowing of the airway caused by scarring.

What are the symptoms?

Noisy breathing, together with difficulty in breathing in, are features of stridor. In severe cases, inadequate oxygen levels in the blood can make the situation life-threatening. Other symptoms depend on the underlying cause. For example, an infection in the voice box may cause a high temperature and a hoarse voice. Any tumor affecting the voice box causes hoarseness, and—if it is malignant—there may be difficulty in swallowing and weight loss.

How is it diagnosed?

The condition is easily diagnosed by listening to the character of the person's breathing. Examination of the voice box with a flexible endoscope identifies the underlying cause. It may be necessary to examine the voice box with the patient under general anesthesia to assess the situation more accurately, especially in children. If a specific lesion is identified, it can be easily biopsied while the individual is anesthetized.

What are the treatment options?

This depends on the underlying cause. Children with laryngomalacia (p. 140) can often be treated before any real problems arise, and the excess floppy tissue can be removed under anesthesia. In cases of stenosis of the voice box, it is possible to widen the narrow part surgically; it may be necessary to carry out a tracheostomy (p. 129) in the interim. Traumatic injury to the voice box often requires surgical intervention, which may also involve a tracheostomy in the first instance. Infection is treated with antibiotics, and in the majority of cases no further treatment is required. Foreign bodies can be removed safely under brief general anesthesia.

Treatment of tumors in the larynx involves removal of the lesion. Benign tumors can often be removed through the mouth. Traditionally, once a malignant tumor was large enough to cause stridor, removal involved a partial or total laryngectomy (removal of the voice box). More recently, removal of cancerous tumors has been carried out successfully through the mouth, using a special laser.

TINNITUS
The sensation of hearing a sound in the absence of any external noise.

Tinnitus is a very common problem, particularly among the elderly. In severe cases, it can become quite disabling.

What is the cause?
Virtually any disease of the external, middle, or inner ear can cause tinnitus. For example, tinnitus occurs with impacted wax, noise-induced hearing loss, Meniere's disease, and, rarely, tumors of the auditory nerve (see Acoustic Neuroma, p. 134, and Otosclerosis, p. 145). It is also associated with a number of conditions including anemia, high blood pressure, and neurological diseases, such as multiple sclerosis, and it can be provoked by medication, including aspirin and some antibiotics.

However, most people who suffer with tinnitus do not have any associated ear disease and in these cases, the underlying cause is not known. Among the theories put forward to explain the problem is that it may be caused by increased or decreased activity in the auditory nerve or by cross stimulation of adjacent nerve fibers within the auditory nerve. Alternatively, it may result from abnormal function of the central processing of auditory information.

What are the symptoms?
Tinnitus can be intermittent or continuous, and its character varies from person to person: It may be heard as a buzzing, humming, or whooshing, among other

Is there a cure for tinnitus?

There is no cure for tinnitus, but some support groups advocate the four Rs as a way of living with and overcoming the condition.

- RECOGNITION A doctor can determine that there is no underlying illness and reassure a patient that the condition is not life threatening and that strategies exist to overcome it.
- RELAXATION Relaxing the body breaks the vicious cycle of tinnitus—worry, tension—tinnitus seems worse—more worry, and so on.
- RETRAINING A sufferer can train his or her mind to become used to tinnitus by listening to other sounds. Taped music played at just below the level of the tinnitus for several hours a day often helps a patient "tune out" the tinnitus.
- RECREATION Keeping physically and mentally active may make tinnitus recede into the background so a sufferer is not conscious of it for long periods of the day.

ASK THE EXPERT

noises. It is usually most noticeable in a quiet environment, especially at night. Tinnitus typically affects both ears, but a single ear can be affected, and in this instance it is important to rule out an underlying cause such as an acoustic neuroma. In most tinnitus patients, the clinical examination is entirely normal. However, the majority have some degree of hearing loss, as confirmed by a hearing test. It is important to find out what sort of impact the tinnitus is having on the individual's life, because this will largely dictate whether or not treatment is required. If there is an underlying medical condition, then the patient may also have symptoms of this condition.

How is it diagnosed?
The diagnosis is made purely on the patient's history because there is no reliable objective method of assessing the intensity of the tinnitus. However, the pitch and the level of noise necessary to obscure the tinnitus can be determined, and this is important for any subsequent treatment. If the tinnitus affects only one ear, a scan of the inner ear is usually carried out to make sure there is not an underlying acoustic neuroma.

What are the treatment options?

Most people suffering with tinnitus require little more than reassurance that there is no sinister underlying problem. Once reassured, many people find that the impact the tinnitus has on their lives is significantly reduced, because they no longer focus on the problem. Simple steps, such as playing soft music in the background at night, are often helpful. Noise generators are available to drown out tinnitus, and some people who use this technique find that the tinnitus remains less noticeable even after the masker is removed. In those people who have significant hearing loss with the tinnitus, a hearing aid may be beneficial because it tends to increase awareness of background noise, making the tinnitus less apparent.

Counseling and relaxation play an important role for people with tinnitus, and a number of self-help groups exist.

What is the outlook?

There is no cure for tinnitus in the majority of cases, but the impact that it has on a person's life can be reduced by appropriate advice and reassurance, together with specific aids or treatments in selected cases.

TONSILLITIS
Inflammation of the tonsils.

The tonsils are situated in the back of the mouth and form part of the ring of glandular tissue that protects the upper gastrointestinal tract and airway from infection. Infection in the tonsils is common, especially in children.

What are the causes?

Allergic patients are more prone to tonsil inflammation. There is generally a bacterial infection, but in some cases the infection is caused by a virus. Streptococcal bacteria may permanently reside deep in the tonsils.

What are the symptoms?

Often, fever and general malaise precede the onset of a sore throat. The sore throat is the predominant symptom, associated with painful, difficult swallowing. There may be an earache and difficulty in opening the mouth. Young children may complain of abdominal pain and may vomit.

The tonsils themselves are swollen and inflamed and there is often pus visible on the surface. There is usually lymph gland swelling in the neck. Occasionally, an abscess may form in the tissues adjacent to the tonsil (see Quinsy, p. 146) and this exacerbates the pain and difficulty in swallowing and opening the mouth.

What are the treatment options?

The mainstay of treatment is pain relief and plenty of fluids. It is not always necessary to give antibiotics, because the disease is usually self-limiting, but in severe cases recovery may be quicker if antibiotics are given. These are available in tablet form, although it may be necessary to give antibiotics and fluids intravenously if the individual is not able to swallow. Generally, symptoms resolve in less than a week. In people who have recurrent infection, removal of the tonsils should be considered. The criteria for tonsillectomy vary, but five episodes a year for more than two years is a reasonable guide.

VERTIGO
Feelings of dizziness and imbalance.

The balance mechanism involves the complex integration of information from several sources, including the semicircular canals in the inner ear, position-sensitive receptors in the arms and legs, and a visual input. These factors are analyzed by the brain, which coordinates balance and movement. A problem at any point can result in vertigo, so it is vital to look at every aspect of the mechanism in order to identify the cause of the problem.

What are the causes?

Disorders of any part of the balance mechanism can result in vertigo. Inner ear damage results from acute viral infection, as in labyrinthitis (p. 138), or from Meniere's disease (p. 140). Similarly, disease of the vestibular nerve can cause vertigo and may, for example, result from a tumor, such as an acoustic neuroma (p. 134). There may be disease in the brain itself as a result of a stroke or tumor or in the spinal cord secondary to multiple sclerosis. There may be disease in the limbs that makes the position receptors no longer work correctly. And it is not only disorders of the balance mechanism itself that can cause dizziness.

Disorders of heart and thyroid function together with other diseases such as anemia can all cause dizziness. In addition, certain drugs can cause dizziness. Even after thorough investigation by doctors, a specific diagnosis is not made in about 30 percent of people.

What are the symptoms?

A wide spectrum of symptoms is included within the term vertigo. Typically, disease of the semicircular canals causes rotational vertigo, in which the person experiences the sensation of the room spinning around him or her. This is often made worse by head movements or by closing the eyes, and in some cases it may be positional. The vertigo may be sudden or gradual in onset and may be constant or intermittent, depending on the cause. The individual may simply feel a sense of imbalance or other nonspecific type of disequilibrium. Depending on the cause of the vertigo, the person may also experience other symptoms originating in the ear. These include hearing loss, tinnitus, and, occasionally, pain or discharge from the ear.

How is it diagnosed?

The vast majority of people are diagnosed on the basis of the history and examination and further investigation is often unnecessary. There is no objective way of reaching a diagnosis in many cases of vertigo. Evidence of disturbance within the balance mechanism can sometimes be seen by observing the eyes (p. 109). People suffering

LIVING WITH VERTIGO

I was in my late 40s when my Meniere's disease started. I began to have spells when I felt the room spinning. They would come on really quickly, but I could usually tell when I was going to have an attack because I'd get a ringing in my right ear just beforehand.

When it's bad, the attacks can last all day, but fortunately that doesn't happen very often. I know some people who have much worse Meniere's disease than I do, and they find it really difficult even to go out sometimes. My hearing tends to be a bit variable as well, although it's never been too much of a problem. I do sometimes worry that it might get worse in the long run, but I have noticed that my symptoms have been much better since I cut out coffee and cut down on the amount of salt I put on my food. I miss having anchovies on my pizza, though! I know there are tablets and even an operation that might help, but at the moment my symptoms aren't too bad and I prefer not to take anything. Hopefully it will stay that way.

from vertigo may also have abnormalities in the way they walk. More detailed assessment of the function of the labyrinth can be performed by looking at the severity and duration of vertigo induced in caloric testing (p. 109).

Intermittent short dizzy spells are likely to be caused by poor function in the semicircular canals. An audiogram is also an important part of the investigative process, because many causes of vertigo that originate in the ear are associated with deafness. Measurement of the electrical activity in the part of the brainstem involved in hearing can be used to identify an acoustic neuroma (p. 134), but more recently this has been replaced by MRI.

What are the treatment options?

This depends on the cause of the vertigo. Most people with vertigo improve with time. The exceptions to this are those people whose problem has a neurological cause, such as an acoustic neuroma or multiple sclerosis. Many people benefit from specific rehabilitative exercises aimed at encouraging the central nervous system to compensate for the damaged part of the balance mechanism.

Numerous medications are available for the treatment of vertigo, but they are often ineffective and may delay the body's natural compensation. There are treatments for the different conditions causing vertigo. For example, in Meniere's disease, an antibiotic to destroy the function of the inner ear is injected into the middle ear. Surgical solutions range from insertion of an ear tube to division of the vestibular nerve supplying the balance organs.

VOCAL CORD PARALYSIS
A condition in which the vocal cords are unable to move.

The larynx serves a number of purposes, including voice production and protecting the lungs from inhalation of saliva or food (aspiration). These functions are made possible by the ability of the vocal cords to open and close when required. If one or both of the cords become immobile, then the individual's lungs are no longer protected from aspiration, the voice will be hoarse and, depending on the position in which the cord is paralyzed, the person can potentially have difficulty breathing.

What are the causes?

The movements of the vocal cords are controlled by tiny muscles, which are stimulated to contract by impulses from the brain carried down through the neck to the larynx in the vagus nerve. The left-sided nerve passes right down into the chest before entering the larynx. Disease affecting any part of this pathway can result in a vocal cord paralysis. A common cause of paralysis is infiltration of the nerve by a tumor, especially in the lung, esophagus, or thyroid gland. In a significant number of people, the nerve becomes damaged during surgery on the neck, particularly thyroid surgery. Some cases may be caused by damage to the nerve during a traffic accident or a sporting injury. Others may result from a neurological disorder such as a stroke. About 15 percent of cases have no attributable cause. Viruses also account for a large number of paralysis cases.

What are the symptoms?
This depends on the position of the vocal cord once paralyzed and whether or not both cords are affected. The most common symptoms of single vocal cord paralysis are hoarseness and an inability to cough adequately. If there is aspiration of food, coughing may follow each mouthful. As a result of foreign material entering the lungs, there is a risk of pneumonia. If both vocal cords are paralyzed, the patient may have difficulty breathing and stridor (p. 151).

How is it diagnosed?
The patient's history gives the first indication of whether or not there is paralysis. The diagnosis is confirmed by examining the larynx using a flexible endoscope. This is performed while the individual is awake, because the vocal cord movements need to be assessed while the person talks. If there is a paralysis, one or both of the cords will not move.

What are the treatment options?
If only one cord is affected and it is fixed in the midline, most people will not require any treatment, because compensation by the other cord takes place over a period of a few months. If one cord is affected and it is fixed in the open position, compensation may take place, but in some instances there may be persistent problems. In this event, the paralyzed cord can be injected with material, usually collagen, in order to push it toward the midline. Alternatively, the cord can be adjusted so that it is positioned closer to the midline.

If there is paralysis of both cords and they are toward the midline, part of one cord can be removed under anesthesia, most often by using a laser. This opens the airway without totally compromising the voice. There are also several operations that pull the cords away from the midline to make the airway wider. These procedures are successful in about two thirds of cases. When both cords are paralyzed in the open position, the larynx becomes incompetent and the person aspirates food and has a very breathy voice. This is rare and treated by tracheostomy (p. 129) to protect the lungs and a laryngectomy (p. 130).

WAX BLOCKAGE
A buildup of wax in the ear canal.

Cerumen, or ear wax, is produced when the output of modified sweat glands in the outer part of the ear canal combines with debris formed by dead skin cells. This wax gradually works its way out toward the pinna as a result of the outward growth of the skin lining the ear canal.

What are the causes?
The amount of wax produced varies considerably from person to person. In some instances, it can cause blockage of the ear canal, particularly in people who have undergone certain types of ear operation—for example, a mastoidectomy, in which the normal anatomical arrangements have been disrupted. However, in the majority of cases, the problem of wax blockage is a result of cleaning the ears with cotton swabs, which can push the wax deep into the ear canal and can traumatize the skin of the ear canal, hampering its outward growth.

What are the symptoms?
People with wax blockage may experience several symptoms, including a sensation of blockage or earache and mild hearing loss. There may also be a dry cough caused by irritation of the vagus nerve, which supplies both the skin of the ear canal and the larynx.

What are the treatment options?
Various agents can soften or dissolve ear wax, ranging from olive oil to baking soda, as well as more specific preparations. They should be instilled into the ear canal with the person lying with the affected ear upward so that the liquid does not run out. If they are not effective, in most situations the ear can be irrigated with warm water by a doctor. If there is an infection or a perforated eardrum, irrigation should not be performed. The alternative is wax clearance by an ENT surgeon who will take care not to cause any problems during removal.

Index

Acknowledgments

Carroll & Brown Limited would also like to thank:

Picture researcher
Julia Hanson

Production manager
Karol Davies

Production controller
Nigel Reed

Computer management
Paul Stradling

Indexer
Jill Dormon

3-D anatomy
Mirashade/Matt Gould

Illustrators
Andy Baker, Jacey, Kevin Jones Associates, Debbie Maizels, Mikki Rain, Halli Verrinder, John Woodcock

Photographers
Jules Selmes, David Murray

Photographic sources
GI = Getty Images; IOL = Institute of Laryngology and Otology, University College London; RNTNE = Royal National Throat Nose & Ear Hospital, Royal Free Hampstead NHS Trust; SPL = Science Photo Library; WTMPL= Wellcome Trust Medical Photographic Library

1 Alfred Pasieka/SPL
6 (left) Secchi-Lecaque/ Roussel-UCLAF/CNRI/SPL
7 Dr Karl Louna/SPL
8 (top left) Mehau Kulyk/SPL
9 GI/Spencer Rowell
10 (top) James Stevenson/SPL
11 (left) GI/Andy Cox
   (right) Photodisc/Doug Menuez
   (bottom right) CNRI/SPL
12 (right) GI/Victoria Blackie
13 Mehau Kulyk/SPL
14 (left) Alfred Pasieka/SPL
   (right) David Murray
18 (bottom left) Alfred Pasieka/SPL
19 (top) Hanan Isachar/Corbis
   (right) David Roberts/SPL
20 (right) CNRI/SPL
21 (bottom) SPL
22 (b. left) Paschal Goetgheluck/SPL
27 (top left) Tony Wright/UCL
28 (bottom) David Murray
29 (bottom) Lauren Shear/SPL

30 (top) Clem Haagner, Gallo Images/Corbis
33 (center right) Secchi-Lecaque/ Roussel-UCLAF/CNRI/SPL
35 (background) Big Pictures
36 (b. right) GI/W & D McIntyre
36-37 GI/Mel Yates
37 (top) GI/John Bragg
   (center) GI/Spencer Rowell
   (bottom) GI/Donovan Reese
38 (left) GI/Joe McBride
   (center) GI/David Chambers
   (right) GI/Michael Dunning
39 GI/Russell Kaye
40 (left) Gail Mooney/Corbis
41 (top right) Carl and Ann Purcell/Corbis
   (center right) Richard Hamilton Smith/Corbis
43 Alfred Pasieka/SPL
44-45 (top) GI/Joe McBride
48 (center) GI/Laurence Monneret
49 (left) Gail Mooney/Corbis
50 Douglas Kirkland/Corbis
55 R. W. Jones/Corbis
56 GI/David Chambers
57 David Murray
58 (bottom) Corbis Stock Market
61 (top) Robert Llewellyn/Corbis
   (b. left) Patrick Bennett/Corbis
   (b. center) Photodisc/Steve Mason
   (b. right) GI/Michael Dunning
68 Tony Arruza/Corbis
72 John Birdsall Photography
73 (top) GI/Rick Rusing
   (bottom) Corbis/Kevin Fleming
75 Corbis Stockmarket
77 John Noble/Corbis
78 Popperfoto/David Joiner
80 (centre) Corbis Stockmarket
   (b. right) Corbis Stockmarket
81 (b. left) Neal Preston/Corbis
   (b. right) GI/Charly Franklin
84 Richard Hamilton Smith/Corbis
85 GI/Chris Rawlings
86 GI/Russell Kaye
90 Courtesy HoMedics UK Ltd.
91 (top) Charles Mauzy/Corbis
   (all others) Eyewire
93 Garden Picture Library/Ron Sutherland/Garden designer Lucy Huntingdon
94 (left) Alfred Pasieka/SPL
   (right) Courtesy Dr. G. Kocjan, University College Hospital, London
95 Andrew Gardner, IOL
98 Alexander Tsiaras/SPL

100-1 AFP/Francois-Xavier Marit
104 Alfred Pasieka/SPL
105 WTMPL
106 Courtesy Karl Storz Endoscopy (UK) Ltd.
107 WTMPL
108 (top) BSIP, Edwige/SPL
109 Charles East, RNTNE
110 BSIP, Edwige/SPL
111 (left) WTMPL
   (right) Charles East, RNTNE
112 (top) CC Studio/SPL
   (inset) Manfred Kage/SPL
   (center left) Chris Priest/SPL
   (center right) Mehau Kulyk/SPL
113 (top) Andrew Gardner, IOL
   (bottom) both Courtesy Dr. G. Kocjan, University College Hospital, London
114 Dr. Karl Louna/SPL
115 (top) Custom Medical Stock/SPL
   (bottom) John Griem/SPL
120 (bottom) CE
121 (left) BSIP, Edwige/SPL
   (centre) Prof. Tony Wright, IOL/SPL
122 (top) John Hadfield/SPL
   (center) Jane Shemilt/SPL
   (bottom) BAHA/Entific Medical Systems
123 (both) James King-Holmes/SPL
124 (top) Charles East, RNTNE
125 (top and center) Andrew Gardner, IOL
   (bottom) Charles East, RNTNE
126 (top) Charles East, RNTNE
   (center) BSIP Boucharlat/SPL
127 Dr. P. Marazzi/SPL
128 Dept. of Clinical Radiology, Salisbury District Hospital/SPL
129 WTMPL
131 Ouellette & Theroux, Publiphoto Diffusion/SPL
132 Tim Beddow/SPL

Thanks
Carroll and Brown would like to thank Dr. Ian H. Flindell, part-time teacher and researcher at the Institute of Sound and Vibration Research at the University of Southampton, England, and independent consultant in subjective acoustics and environmental noise.